Samantha X is Amanda Goff, former journalist and mother of two.

Amanda started her career as a reporter for London's tabloid press before moving to Australia for sun, sea and sex.

After 13 years as a magazine writer in Sydney, Amanda decided selling sex was far more fun and lucrative, and that the stories she heard from within the brothel's walls were more fascinating than any exclusive she covered.

Amanda outed herself as a high-class escort on national television, causing a public outcry. Her story about being an 'escort mum' went global, garnering many supporters – and critics – around the world.

She now combines her two loves: sex and writing, as the sex editor of *Penthouse* magazine, while also playing agony aunt to the hundreds of men and women who write to her at www.samanthax.com.au

She lives by the beach with her two children.

HOOKED

THE SALACIOUS SECRETS OF SAMANTHA X: SYDNEY'S TOP HIGH-CLASS CALL GIRL

SAMANTHA X

EBURY
PRESS

An Ebury Press book
Published by Random House Australia Pty Ltd
Level 3, 100 Pacific Highway, North Sydney NSW 2060
www.randomhouse.com.au

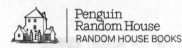

Penguin
Random House
RANDOM HOUSE BOOKS

First published by Ebury Press in 2014
This edition published by Ebury Press in 2015

Random House Books is part of the Penguin Random House group of companies whose
addresses can be found at global.penguinrandomhouse.com.

National Library of Australia
Cataloguing-in-Publication Entry

Samantha X, author.
Hooked / Samantha X.

ISBN 978 0 85798 448 7 (paperback)

Prostitutes–New South Wales–Sydney–Biography.
Prostitution–New South Wales–Sydney.
Brothels–New South Wales–Sydney.

306.742092

Cover design by Blue Cork
Front cover photograph © Juanmonino/Getty Images
Back cover photograph © Fabrizio Lipari
Typeset in Minion Pro by Midland Typesetters, Australia
Printed in Australia by Griffin Press, an accredited ISO AS/NZS 14001:2004
Environmental Management System printer

Random House Australia uses papers that are natural, renewable and recyclable products and
made from wood grown in sustainable forests. The logging and manufacturing processes are
expected to conform to the environmental regulations of the country of origin.

Contents

To those who take the road less travelled . . .
and bloody enjoy it.

Chapter One

SAMANTHA

Client X

Client X was not like most of my clients. What I mean is that he was gorgeous. His eyes were blue, his hair sandy, streaked blond by the sun no doubt, while surfing, and his arms were perfect. Arms are so important, aren't they? Too big and he's a steroid muncher, too skinny and he can hardly hold a cup of tea, let alone your panting body. But from the moment we locked eyes in the 'intro' room and he chose me, I felt my tummy do a backflip. This man was paying $450 for the hour to have sex with me. Shouldn't I be paying him? I thought, smiling wryly to myself as we walked up the red velvet stairs to one of the decadently themed boudoir rooms.

I am a hooker, escort, working girl. Whatever you want to call it, they all mean the same thing: I sell my body for money. Shock horror! It seems quite the rage these days, doesn't it? You've read the books – *The Secret Diary of a London Call*

Girl, Manhattan Call Girl. I saw in my local bookshop there's even a *Brazilian Call Girl* ... well, g'day everyone, here's another addition to your worldwide map; I am your Sydney call girl.

My working name is Samantha. My place of employment was a brothel or, as it preferred to be called, a five-star boutique establishment called The Bordello. (Not its real name, but ask any working girl or client and they'll tell you where I mean, except – silly me! Who is going to identify themselves to you as either one of those?)

Not just any run-of-the-mill brothel, The Bordello was a mighty fine one. In fact, I would go as far to say I was working at Sydney's finest, a colourful place with clients that included CEOs, celebrities, sportsmen and affluent businessmen, as well as hot tradies and 18-year-old surfers who had saved up for months for the upscale experience. Men didn't just come from all over the country to visit, they came from all over the *world*: America, Canada, France, Germany, Japan ... and not just men, either. Girls from France, Italy and Spain would travel here, spend a few months working and fly home armed with a bundle of cash.

Clients would marvel at the décor and go gaga over the girls, knowing that, while the prices were a little on the steep side, you got what you paid for. And they would always, always come back for more.

'There is no place quite like this place, honey,' drawled an American pastor dressed in a Hawaiian shirt, as he masturbated on my stomach. 'And certainly not one that is legal.'

Its reputation as the world's finest bordello was firmly set in sparkling gold, and the girls who made it so knew they were working in the best sex-selling, money-making safest cleanest establishment there is. Did I like my job? *I bloody loved it.*

'It's my birthday today,' my client smiled shyly. 'I'm 29.' As he took off his clothes, revealing a tanned, fit body, with a beautifully carved tattoo of a dragon on his perfect back, he looked in pretty good shape to me. He pulled me closer, so close I could feel his breath on my face, smell his manly scent mixed in with aftershave, what was it? I was getting so good at this game . . . Calvin Klein? Dior Homme?

Who cares, I thought dreamily as I pulled him closer, quickly scanning the room. Condoms, check. Lube, check. Tummy sucked in, legs apart, wet pussy, check check *check*.

'Fuck I need this,' he groaned as he tugged at my panties. Usually at this stage, I quietly grab the lube when the client isn't noticing, my fingers quickly wetting my pussy, purring, 'I'm so wet, baby,' to stroke his fragile ego. No need to fake this one. This client, his name, what was it, Scott? Sean? It didn't matter. He was fucking gorgeous.

Pulling at my lace, he forced my legs open, exposing my wet, swollen clit. 'Can I?' he asked, going to lick me.

'Oh of course, darling,' I breathed. 'I want it, I need it . . . be filthy with me . . .'

I lay back, smiling, as his warm tongue explored the creases and folds of my pussy, licking, sucking, tasting me. Wow. I grabbed his sandy hair, pushed his head further inside, closer . . .

He grabbed my lube and took his cock in one hand, then started to rub along the shaft. I watched as he grew harder. 'Start sucking, babe,' he moaned. I grabbed a condom, slid it on his throbbing cock with my mouth, a skill only working girls learn to perfect. Before long he was plunging his hard throbbing cock inside me. Urgent, forceful even, deeper and deeper.

Holy shit, I thought, watching him in the mirror as he flipped me over, hands all over me, plunging his cock again and again into my wetness. How lucky am I?

'Fuck, here it comes,' he panted, and gripped my arse, pinning me down while I could feel his cock explode, pulsating inside me. I watched his face while he came. I always like to do this with my clients, more so for comedy value at the imitation heart-attack expressions I have witnessed. But this one was expressionless. You know how they say sharks have dead eyes? I suppose it was a bit like that.

Client X was far away, I could tell. The sex, while enjoyable for me, seemed mechanical for him, and his mind was in a different place. I felt he was going through the motions because he was here, in Sydney's finest brothel, and he'd paid for the hour, it was his birthday and he was going to enjoy it. But something wasn't quite right.

As a woman who meets many men a day, I learn to read them pretty quickly. James Bond has nothing on me, the skills I've learnt. A quick scan of his clothes while he's in the shower, or the way he arranges his effects, for example, usually tells me what kind of man he is. I can read a man from his clothes, neatly folded (meticulous, a clean freak), and from the way he folds his socks (too much time in front of the computer – an internet nerd?).

I have one regular who arranges his watch, wallet and phone ensemble all so neatly, you could swear he had measured it with a ruler to make it a perfectly straight line. His job? An aeronautical engineer, of course. He paid attention to detail. He noticed if I had a tiny rip in my stockings, or whether my eye make-up had changed. He liked lingerie kept on (my body not his) and he carefully tweaked and caressed my nipples until erect as if he was fine-tuning the inner mechanics of the new Boeing Dreamliner 787.

But back to my troubled client. I wanted to try to get to the bottom of it. 'Beer?' I offered, opening the fridge (all rooms came with a free minibar). We still had around 40 minutes left on the clock and, while young good-looking clients usually have somewhere else to be and don't like to hang around, I had a feeling Client X would stay. He was in no rush to open the door to his real life again.

He lit a cigarette, took one long drag and exhaled slowly, puffing out those smoke rings only a certain type of smoker can do. The way the rings curl into the air perfectly always transfixes me momentarily.

'So what else are you doing today, Birthday Boy?' I asked, trying to act casual but hoping this would lead to a glimpse into his life.

'Not much,' he replied, taking another drag. 'My wife has something arranged, I dunno. Something with the kids.'

I glanced at his hand. No ring, but they usually took it off when they came here. Guilt? He was 29, and had said kids, plural. He'd obviously got married when he was young, maybe too young, and was feeling what, maybe trapped?

'Marriage is hard work, isn't it?' I replied, getting up to make myself a drink. Men quite often feel more comfortable talking to my back sometimes: less eye contact, less confrontation. Or maybe they just like staring at my arse. Whatever the reason, my backside has heard many a confession. Thank God men aren't big talkers – clenching my buttocks for more than two minutes isn't comfortable.

'Yeah, I just don't know what to do. I love her but, y'know, I'm not just in love with her any more. But those kids. Man, I'd do anything for those kids.'

I closed my eyes. Another sad marriage. Was there any other type? I felt for this man, so young and feeling like this already. For the rest of our time together I lay in his arms and listened while he talked and talked. About how he knew his marriage was over, but how he felt shame and disappointment from hurting his kids and his wife. He had never spoken about his feelings before, he told me, but somehow, here in this room with me naked, my breasts pressed up on his chest and my pussy still throbbing from the force of his cock, I could tell he felt safe.

'I don't want to admit the dream is broken,' he said sadly, looking away. Was that a tear in his eye? I glanced at him, knowing exactly what he meant. While it had been two years since Luke and I separated, it was always going to be my sad story. My failure.

'I know,' I replied, stroking his arms. 'It's like finding out Father Christmas doesn't exist.' The disbelief, the crashing disappointment. No happy fat man delivering presents with the help of elves wearing little turned-up shoes? Nope, and no happily ever after, either.

I told him briefly about myself, about leaving an unhappy marriage, but with two beautiful babies I didn't want to hurt.

'My kids have blossomed since we split,' I reassured him. 'There's no more tension. Mummy's happy and Daddy's happy. Sometimes, the grass *is* greener on the other side, just remember that.'

I felt despair for this man. This young, handsome man,

full of promise and life, was, underneath, struggling, battling internal turmoil and guilt over whether to leave his wife or not. He hadn't come for sex. He'd come to unburden.

'Hey thanks for that,' he said afterwards, buttoning up his shirt. 'Sometimes it really helps to talk to a stranger. I wouldn't tell my closest friends what I've told you.'

I know, I thought. I'd heard it so many times. So many.

In my 'real life', I am a 39-year-old journalist. I say 'real life' or 'outside world' a lot in this job because here, in the Emperor's Suite or the King's Castle room, with the splashing marble water features, blurry scenes of exchanging of $100 notes and black credit cards, quick urgent fucks with strangers, and an intercom buzzing 'Time's up', this is a far, far cry from my real life. And there's one thing I want to stress: these two worlds, Samantha's and Amanda's, never, ever collide.

Samantha never gatecrashes Amanda's safe, normal world. And Amanda tries her best not to appear in Samantha's bookings. I want to make it crystal shiny see-through clear before we embark on this journey that I do not, nor will ever, work at home. Men do not come back to my house. They don't even know where I live, and most do not know my real name. I work the weeks my children are with their father and the brothel is a good 20-minute drive from my home. When I'm a mum, I'm a mum, and when my kids are safely tucked away with their father for the week, and it's time to slip on the suspenders and stockings, I am Samantha. When I say the worlds never collide, they are not even in the same stratosphere.

But Amanda, bless her, can't help peek her head in during Samantha's appointments. Her world is so much more exciting!

I try hard to be a different person with Samantha, but sometimes I let the real me come out. I rarely lie. Words that are untrue feel like barbed wire coming out of my mouth. Even my therapist, Doris, once kindly advised me to 'learn how to lie.'

While most working girls invent something ridiculous when a client asks what their real job is (one English backpacker told clients she bred miniature horses for a living; not true, of course, but sounds far more interesting than studying social work), I often give them edited glimpses into my life.

I did decide to tell a select few of my clients about this book, and wow, did I find out who has the egos! Most wanted a starring role, funnily enough even the married ones. 'Sure, you can use me,' a heart surgeon grunted as he stuck two of his fingers in my pussy, his cold gold wedding band pressing against my swollen lips. 'You can even use my first name. But please, Samantha, say I am good in bed.' Another client, a young, confident, sexy Lebanese builder told me I could put his photo in.

'But I want a whole chapter dedicated to me, babe, not just a few lines,' he said earnestly, racking up several lines of cocaine he brought with him on a mirror.

As a reporter – a hack – I have spent years interviewing people about subjects they don't want to talk about. I was used to making people sweat (for the wrong reasons) until publication date.

My skill, though, remains the same: extracting information from people in a subtle way. And in my newfound career that skill came in very handy indeed. I knew how to make men talk, to feel comfortable with me. And when they felt comfortable with me, they told me things 'they'd never told anyone before'. Once that bond was created, I knew that not only did I help them with their issue, but also that they would probably be back for more. Hey, just call me the 'tart with a heart'!

You do realise the biggest myth about men and prostitutes, don't you? They don't really come for the sex, not all of them. It's the intimacy they crave, the closeness. There is a reason men are happy to pay an extra $50 to kiss, why they nervously request the 'girlfriend experience' while clutching your hand more than the 'pornstar experience'. Not one client has asked me for porn sex but 99 per cent have asked whether I would kiss and cuddle them. Surprised?

In fact, the kinkiest thing anyone has requested of me was from a gentle, caramel-coloured, exotic-looking IT specialist. Late twenties, married, nice full lips. 'Excuse me, Samantha,' he said shyly while unclipping my suspender belt. 'Could you possibly pretend to be my mother-in-law today?' Cheeky bastard – did I look that old?

So, sorry. I know this is terribly worrying for women and rather a relief for men. But I am about to shatter your pointy-fingered perceptions. Instead of assuming that sex in brothels is disgusting, pornographic, depraved and repulsive, and that men who go there are monsters or perverts, fuelled by a need to rape or dominate, or are just plain losers, and the women who work there are victims of some sort – junkies, dumb, can't get any other job, or would do anything for a dollar, or that we all have mental issues – you'll soon see that it's more complicated than that.

I am a mum, someone's daughter, an ex-wife and a journalist. I'm not a junkie and I prefer early mornings and exercise to late nights and drugs. I am not a model, either; I am attractive and look after my body, but it's nothing seriously amazing. I own my own house in one of Sydney's most affluent suburbs.

My ex-husband is a successful businessman. My parents are upper middle class. I went to private school and graduated from university with a Bachelor of Arts (Honours) degree. I chose to be a hooker. And though many similar books out there are all about how degrading and disempowering the sex industry is, I disagree wholeheartedly.

I hadn't just found a novel job to pay the bills; I'd found my *calling.*

What makes me different from other women? Well, I love sex, but I got sick of doing it for free with men who promised the earth and delivered mud. I love getting paid to do what I enjoy. I also love being in control and feeling empowered. You want me to kiss you? Sure, that's $50. You want me to dress up as a nurse? Open your wallet. You want to have sex with me, no ties? You don't want to go for coffee dates or pretend to like my kids? You just want to get laid? Thanks for your honesty – and that's $450 please.

Some say that my life isn't real. That what goes on in bordellos is a fantasy. In truth it's more realistic than RSVP. I don't want to hear your bullshit on what movies you like, and I'm sure deep down you don't give a shit about my music collection. Let's get dirty. Then you can leave.

As a 'lady of the night', I work the days and weeks and hours I choose to work. There's no boss raising their eyebrows when I leave early to pick my kids up, or calling me into a meeting dead on 6 pm knowing I have two little people in after-school care counting on me.

I love taking January and February off to be with my babies in the summer holidays, instead dumping them at vacation care in order to work. I love looking forward to the Easter break and the summer holidays because that means long, delicious days with my kids without the phone ringing, without emails firing at me, without being wracked with guilt ('I should be in the office . . .').

Before I face the wrath of other working mums, I do realise that most women don't have a choice. Of course I don't believe that working makes you a bad parent. You're setting a great example to your kids by working. And Jesus, a coffee is $4 these days. Who doesn't need to work?

But I do think being happy makes you a happy parent. And I know I am deliriously happy.

It's not as though I haven't earned my dues. I've been a magazine writer for close to 20 years now. I know what hard work is like. I know what office life is like. I know deadlines. I've had tricky editors. I've signed enough contracts to know about commitment and being part of a team. But I've done my time. I climbed the ladder – and you know what? The view wasn't that great when I got to the top. The closer I got to being the boss, the further away I was getting from what I really wanted: freedom and family.

Life is about choice – freedom of choice. Rightly or wrongly, I choose to live this way.

I don't have the luxury of being a stay-at-home mum, spending my overworked husband's money. I don't have a family to support me, to mind the kids while I nip out. My family live in Europe and I have more in-depth conversations with my local barista than with my parents.

It's me, myself and I. It always has been.

Samantha gives me financial security, and I no longer have sex with men for free. I just can't be bothered.

So who are my clients? The men who pay almost $500 for 60 minutes of my time are pretty normal: 80 per cent are married, and 20 per cent would love to find true love. (Sounds like the 80 per cent need to have a serious chat with my 20 per cent about the reality of 'true love'!)

The men I see are your husbands, partners, bosses, work colleagues, brothers and sons. Happily married men come, unhappily married men come, single men, party guys, health freaks. There is no type. That guy on the train? Maybe. The barista making your coffee? Hmmm, probably his boss. Your intimidating manager? For sure. Hey, I put him in a better mood for you! Your husband? Um . . . next question!

But honestly, yes darling, maybe even your husband. Feeling a bit uneasy? Admit it, there is that niggling doubt. Where was he that time, drinking till 2 am on a Monday night? Why was his phone turned off during the day for a few hours? You haven't had sex in weeks, or has it been a few months now . . . but that's fine, he hasn't got a sex drive these days, has he? I'm not saying all men would, but a lot do. There is a reason this bordello makes a fortune day in, day out, 24 hours a day, seven days a week, and only shuts Christmas Day. It's called supply and demand. Men demand, we supply. And there's an awful lot of demanding going on – an awful lot of unsatisfied men out there.

Hey! We know about you, darling! We all know about unsatisfied women – it's all women talk about. To each other, in magazines, on TV talk shows. *How to have it all!* We want the career, the kids, the marriage, the body, the wrinkle-free face. The world knows about the needs of women, we never bloody shut up about them.

But what about men?

Their needs are a little more basic. They just want to feel loved. And they feel loved through sex. It really is as simple as that.

Samantha

Let's be honest. When was the last time you and your husband held each other, naked, in bed? When was the last time you let him go down on you without wincing or mentally making a to-do list of all your chores tomorrow? When was the last time you kissed him – properly kissed him – your tongue exploring his? Or listened to his problems and worries without thinking, 'Yeah, well, what about me?'?

Stop. Stop there for a minute. Stop the rage bubbling inside at me. I know what you're thinking: 'How dare she say that I should listen to his problems when I've had three screaming kids all day'.

I know it's hard with kids around. I'm a mother myself, remember? I was one of those women who would push my husband away. I felt too tired, too fat, too hairy. But if you let your sex life slip, you're probably going to make another hooker a few hundred bucks. Not *your* husband of course, no he wouldn't do that, would he? I'm talking about other women's husbands, partners and boyfriends, of course.

He is the man, and he has a duty to provide for you and the family. But you have a duty, too. Did you forget that? Men need sex. Call it primal, selfish, whatever you want, but stop burying your head in the sand. I hear it time and time and time again: 'I adore my wife but she never wants sex' . . . 'she seems to be asexual' . . . 'she doesn't want me any more' . . . 'she's a good mother, but not affectionate to me'.

Is that you he's talking about? It doesn't have to be every day, or even every few days. Once a week, maybe. I see men whose wives haven't put out for months, even years, and I'm sorry women, but what the fuck do you expect your husband to do? Wank in the shower for the rest of his life?

He doesn't care if you've put on a few kilos or need a wax. Hell, he won't even notice! He loves you, he really does, and he just wants to put his cock in his wife's pussy.

I've lost count of the number of times men have admitted to me they would prefer to have sex with their wives than me; it's just that they've given up with them. 'I would much rather spend this money on my wife, taking her out for dinner, going back to a hotel, than coming here. It's just that she's lost interest in me,' a client told me once, just after he'd cum on my tits. 'No offence though, Samantha . . .'

'None taken,' I replied, and genuinely meant it. My opinion of him had just gone up. If only his wife knew how he felt about her. So please listen to me, ladies. I know what I'm talking about.

Don't get upset with me. I'm not making this up. I spend hours with men, locked up together in one room for sometimes five or six hours, naked and terribly vulnerable. I see a side to them they would never show even their closest friends, even you. Confessions, confusions, tears, admissions of guilt, secret drug habits, secret sex lives, hidden desires. Don't pretend this world doesn't exist because I am telling you, woman to woman, it does. *I live in it.*

I know what pricks men can be. God, they're selfish. While they are basic creatures, a bit like panting, dribbling dopey dogs, they are bloody selfish. I'll never forget the 'stressed' and 'exhausted' shoe-shop manager who wanted to wank in my pussy during his lunch break before nodding off for half an hour. 'My wife has just given birth to twin boys,' he said moodily, after waking. 'I didn't realise how exhausting it can be. I just haven't had a full night's sleep since they were born.' I had to bite my tongue. What about her, you selfish prick?

Sometimes I tell these men to get their act together, too. Is there a reason your wife doesn't want sex? Don't just nudge your dick in her back as she's about to nod off. Give her a little shoulder rub, listen to her day, take the bins out, help her with the kids, and then, yeah, you may get rewarded. Of course, I don't want to advise them too much – I might talk myself out of a job!

Take one of my regulars, Peter, an older gentleman, with kind eyes hiding behind sensible spectacles. He books me every three weeks or so for two hours, and in that time he massages my back and feet before he slips his hard cock into my pussy from behind. A few frantic thrusts and then he comes all over my nicely massaged and relaxed back. 'My wife never lets me massage her,' he whispered once in my ear. 'She doesn't like the oil all over the sheets.' I couldn't really blame her. At least I didn't have to do the laundry at the brothel. But all he wanted to do with a woman was to massage her back, to give her pleasure. Was a tiny bit of oil really that much of a problem? Did Peter's wife know he had been paying to massage women for over 15 years? If she was aware, did she actually care? I wondered. Was she perhaps even relieved someone else was fucking her husband and getting their sheets dirty instead of hers?

No, men aren't the tough creatures we think they are. I have seen men from all walks of life, from the hardest of criminals – men who have bullet wounds for Christ's sake – to the ball-breaking suits who run some of the country's top businesses. I have seen them all, nude and raw, and at their most honest. And the one thing they all have in common? They don't understand women. They want to please them, but don't really know how. And, of course, men all want to feel loved.

But more importantly than that, they have a lot of love to give and want to give it. It just so happens that I am the messenger. And what, my friends, is so bloody wrong with that?

AMANDA

Wish you were here . . .

Losing your virginity is supposed to shape the way you perceive sex in your adult life. Isn't that what they say? What can I tell you about my experience? The one thing I took from that drunken fumble on a rock by the beach in Sorrento, Italy is that 25 years later, the smell of Jack Daniel's still makes me gag.

I was 15 and on holiday with my parents and younger sister. The hotel was probably one of the best in Italy. I remember the white, sparkling, sweeping staircase that led to the magnificent gardens, the two pools where we spent our days and the upmarket terrace where dark, swarthy waiters dressed like penguins would serve us dinners of creamy pasta, white melt-in-your-mouth fish and sugary tiramisu. I came from a good family. My father was one of London's respected businessmen and my mother was a conservative yet glamorous daughter of the Middle Eastern elite.

Holidays like this were the norm for our family. We were treated to the good life – my father, an East End boy done good, was determined to give us kids the things in life he was never privileged to. And to his credit, he never forgot his roots. We were never allowed to take anything for granted.

'I take you all to the best places in the world,' he said, 'because I never want any man to think that you will be impressed if and when he does it for you.'

He also once said, 'There's always going to be someone younger and prettier than you,' and that's advice I'll take to my grave, too.

It wasn't so much the hotel that impressed me. A family of London-born Italians who were also holidaying at the same resort had caught my eye. The Pintos: extremely wealthy coffee importers, and in particular, Gianni Pinto, their 15-year-old son. Gianni wasn't much to look at, a bit tubby and sweaty, but he smelt nice and expensive and, more importantly, he seemed to take an interest in me. I noticed the way he stared as I got out of the pool. I knew when my nipples stuck out, pushing against my bikini top, he was watching, smiling. And I felt something I hadn't really felt before – a dampness between my legs, a tummy-swirling, leg-crossing feeling I wasn't used to. Desire.

When Gianni asked whether he could take me for a walk one evening, I was beside myself with excitement and nerves.

'I want you back in your hotel room by 9 pm,' said my mother. I wore my best holiday clothes, a long, floaty, floral skirt with a little singlet and heels. I wasn't sure what I was dressing for, but looking back, I was ridiculously overdressed for a walk on the beach.

I remember Gianni was wearing a black T-shirt, blue jeans and heavy black cowboy boots. He'd brought with him not only his lanky brother Franco, but also a bottle of Jack Daniel's. We each took swigs from it, sitting on the rock, watching the sun go down, the rays gently dancing on the waves. I wasn't a drinker – I'd never touched neat alcohol, so a few gulps of whisky, plus too much sun mixed with nerves, was a recipe for disaster.

The next thing I remember is lying down on the rock with a heaving, sweating Gianni on top of me, and my nice floaty skirt hoisted up by my hips.

'Can I?' he panted, nudging his hard naked penis into the top of my thigh, his cowboy boots digging into my ankles. 'I said, can I?'

Everything started to spin. The sun had gone down, and I could hear the waves crashing against the rocks, the smell of sea salt mixed with Jack Daniel's on his breath.

'What?' I slurred, drunk, unable to fathom what was really happening. I blinked, trying to focus. How did I end up on my back? Franco was standing over us laughing, rubbing his crotch, his eyes beady, his lips curled up with his tongue licking either side.

Nausea was swirling inside me, my head was spinning – what the fuck was happening?

Did I say yes, did I consent? I don't remember. But I can still feel the pain even now, the searing pain inside, as if I was being ripped in two while Gianni heaved and panted on top of me, his cock opening up my pussy, stretching it for the first time, and then the feeling of warm blood as it trickled down my leg.

I remember the burning humiliation, the embarrassment as Franco and Gianni walked off, laughing at me together. 'Did you like losing your *cherry*?' Franco called out to me.

Wait. That was sex? I somehow fumbled my way back to the hotel. I swung open the door to the room I was sharing with my younger sister, who looked up in shock at my dishevelled state.

'I think I just lost my virginity,' I slurred, before running to the bathroom and throwing up in the toilet.

'You're disgusting,' she sneered at me, and went back to bed. I spent the night asleep on the bathroom floor in the foetal position, waking only to vomit what was now just a dark-coloured liquid, pure Jack Daniel's.

Of course back at school I became the second coolest girl in class for being the second girl in the year to lose her virginity. It was a big kudos for me, until my mum found out. A friend's mother had called her to tell her.

Mum's face was white when I came home from school one afternoon. I thought someone had died. 'Amanda, is it true? Is it true that this . . . this . . . *thing* happened while we were on holiday?' she wailed, her eyes searching mine for answers.

I nodded, welling up too. Despite my teenage bravado at getting laid, the incident had left me confused and feeling dirty. Was this my chance to talk to her about sex?

She closed her eyes for a second, as if trying to gather her thoughts, some words. 'You *slut*. My daughter is a slut,' she whispered in shock. 'How could you do this to me? You slut, Amanda. Did you get paid for it? Tell me, did you get paid for it?' The fury and disgust was written all over her face, and the shame and confusion burned inside me. *I was a slut, I should have got paid for it.*

20

Amanda

Mum didn't talk to me for a week – and sex was never mentioned in our house again. Not that it had ever been mentioned before that. But the words stuck. I was only 15, and while I didn't know much about sex, I learnt two things: 1) It was dirty and 2) you could get paid for it.

Chapter Two

SAMANTHA
Pump up the volume

There is a man who comes to fuck me every few weeks. He brings his own stereo. 'I can't stand the music at this place,' he told me on our first encounter. He calls himself Joe, but we both know that isn't his real name. Joe is one of my more quirky clients; I like him a lot. He's handsome and Italian, a fierce Catholic, and he has lots of money. What he does for work I'm never quite sure, something in banking I think. He wears Hugo Boss suits, Italian leather shoes and has these amazing green eyes, which I find very sexy with his sweet-smelling exotic skin.

Joe is one of my married clients. He has three young kids and a stressful job, yet he seems to find the time to visit our brothel regularly.

Joe likes me to lick and suck his balls while I wank him off. It's quite tricky to get the position right with this request, as I always like to have one eye on my client's face to note his expressions, just to make sure he doesn't look bored rigid. His wife, he says, doesn't fuck anymore. 'We haven't had sex in six months,' he tells me. 'When I try, she scolds me and pushes me away. I've just given up. I'm not sure she even finds me attractive anymore, or likes me for that matter.'

But Joe will never leave his wife, not because he doesn't want to, but being a staunch Catholic, divorce is not an option. 'It would kill my parents and no matter what anybody says, children are affected by divorce and I can't put them through that.'

Today, Joe didn't bring his music. 'Just get me a gin and tonic please, darling,' he said, peeling off his tie. 'A strong one.'

'No music today, Joe?' I smiled, clinking ice into a glass.

'I don't feel like music,' he replied. 'I'm stressed, Samantha. I'm in big shit and I don't know what to do. You're the only person I can tell.'

'What's up?' I asked, handing him his drink. I sat down beside him on the bed and rolled down my stockings.

'I'm being blackmailed. This bitch is threatening to tell my wife about our affair if I don't give her $200,000.'

Affair? Another woman?

'What?' I stammered. 'A girl from here, this brothel, is blackmailing you?' For a second I felt a twinge of ridiculous jealousy – was Joe fucking another girl here?

'I met her on this website for sugar daddies,' he explained. 'I paid her, gave her cash, about $700 per meeting, and we had sex. I paid for her new nose, tits, Botox and teeth, and now she wants a car and her loan paid off. I decided to call the whole thing off and the greedy cow is now blackmailing me. Fuck, Samantha, she knows my address. Her mother lives in the next friggin' street.'

'Jesus, Joe,' I replied, shaking my head. I wasn't sure what shocked me most – the fact that this woman had stooped so low, or the fact that Joe was on some sugar-daddy website. Where did he find the time for all of this?

Aha! Those famous words. 'My husband would never cheat on me – he doesn't have *the time*.'

How often have we uttered those words with such conviction? I used to say it too. But believe me – they find the time. I've had very important businessmen call their wives, while they are naked with their stiff cocks in my mouth, to tell them they're in a meeting and won't be home till late. One client, an advertising exec, actually insists on calling his blonde media-friendly wife pretty much as soon as we enter the room. 'I'll pick you up from the office at 4.30, darling,' he says earnestly to her as he cock-slaps my greased-up tits. While the danger obviously turns him on, I can't help feel a bit guilty. That poor, unsuspecting woman. She's probably a lovely person. I can imagine her waiting at the office, timing when to put on her lip gloss, getting ready for her doting husband.

Joe was naked now, on the bed, with drink number two well underway.

'Do you think I should give her the money? Just to get rid of her? The last one wanted $6000 to go away, which was fine, but $200,000? I'm not that rich anymore, Sam.'

Hang on, the 'last one'?

So it turns out Joe not only visits me every few weeks, but he has at least five or six 'sugar babes' on the go, too. The deal with this website is that it's a bit like RSVP except the man has to pay for the woman either by giving her a monthly allowance or paying her per visit, which Joe prefers to do. A visit may include dinner, drinks and sex – no strings attached.

And don't you dare call these women prostitutes – Joe said they get *very* offended. 'They can pick and choose who they fuck,' Joe explained, sharing a mocking smile with me.

'Joe, why bother with them? Why not just come here? At least you know we're not going to blackmail you.'

I wasn't offering him false comfort. Sex in brothels is safe. When I say safe, I mean we meet, we fuck, you leave. The actor Charlie Sheen once said about prostitutes: 'I don't pay hookers for sex. I pay them to leave.'

No exchanging of phone numbers (you'd get sacked), no risk of texts in the middle of the night, and certainly no risks of falling in love and getting hurt. Not to mention condoms for everything, even oral, plus regular STI checks for women who work there.

Why was a smart man like Joe, who had a lot to lose if his wife ever found out, taking such a stupid risk with this website?

'Because while I love coming here, Samantha, and the sex and the company are great, I hate the buzzer that goes off to tell me I have five minutes to get out. It just reminds me I'm in a brothel. I want a relationship. To go out for dinner, have a lovely evening and to feel like I have a girlfriend.'

Joe clearly likes to fuck a variety of pussies. But it's not enough. He wants the full-on girlfriend experience – that tummy-tingly feeling you get when you're about to go on a date with someone you don't know that well – the new smells, new sparkly conversation, someone else's touch. For men, the experience of coming to a brothel or having a bit of side, is far, far more than cock in pussy, insert ten times (if you're lucky) before blowing. Repeat after me: it's not about cock, it's about connection.

But Joe's predicament had me stumped. How much more complicated did he need to make his life? Imagine living in fear that some woman was going to tell all to your poor wife.

'Of course you shouldn't pay the money, Joe,' I said, running my fingers along his back, caressing the ripples of his muscles. 'Can't you go to a lawyer or something? Maybe the cops?'

'I did that already,' he replied glumly. 'I asked the police officer if a woman was hypothetically blackmailing a married man, what should he do?'

'And?'

'The officer winked at me and said, "Who's been a naughty boy then?" It's not worth going down that path. It's too dangerous, I'll be too exposed.'

Poor, silly Joe. Nobody wants to be the one to say 'I told you so', but there are a couple of reasons brothels make so much money. Anonymity and ease. For starters, we are completely confidential about our clients. And while some, like Joe, crave the 'girlfriend experience', others just want a guaranteed lay. 'Why should I spend a few hundred bucks on a woman on a date and still not even get a kiss?' a client remarked once. You can see his point. Women are hard work. We don't make it easy for a man to approach us. We can be stand-offish and pouty. I don't blame men for wanting it all to be a bit easier.

Working girls aren't greedy, either. Not all of us. I rarely accept tips (believe it or not that makes me feel like a hooker in a negative way) – unless they're a Yank. I once tried to turn down a $350 tip but the Californian was so insulted I ended up reluctantly stuffing the notes into my bag. It still somehow felt like stealing.

I don't hustle, that is, trying to work it so that the client extends his stay in the room. These men are already paying top dollar to be here. Why take the piss? I want my clients to leave feeling elated and content, not ripped off.

There was a dear, dull client, Tom, who would pay $600 an hour for me to come to his hotel room every two weeks. Our three hours were spent watching the AFL, then the cricket, then listening to a few of his racist jokes while I ate the Pringles from the minibar. (I'd leave him five bucks for the crisps – we all know how over-priced hotel minibars are.) It was the same every time – even the same hotel room, with me sitting on the huge king-size bed in my lingerie, Tom in greying Y-fronts, his eyes glued to the TV, my eyes glued to the alarm clock by the side of the bed, mentally checking over every time the digits moved: 180 minutes to go, 179 minutes . . .

If I ever so much as tried to kiss him, Tom would push me away gently. 'Maybe next time, Samantha,' he'd murmur, his eyes not leaving the TV screen. At first I was confused, even a bit hurt. Maybe I wasn't his type. Did he ask for petite and blonde and get stuck with tall and brunette? Was I the wrong side of 30, but he was too kind to tell the agency?

The other girls had told me he was like this. 'Oh, lucky you!' exclaimed Amy, a striking, tall, well-read, well-travelled Kiwi. She was one of my favourite girls whom I worked with. 'He's a great client, so easy. We just sit there and discuss politics and exchange our travel stories. He never wants sex, just the company. He'll see you for a few months, then go onto someone else.'

But this wasn't so easy for me.

Though Tom wouldn't hurt a fly, I found our meetings painful. I hated AFL with a passion, almost as much as cricket. At least if there was sex it would kill, oh a minute or two, maybe? But no. He simply wanted his own version of the 'girlfriend experience' – the kind of girlfriend who lay in bed watching sport on TV and doing not much else. I don't know many girlfriends who would be able to do that for so long without hurling something at the screen.

My first ever appointment with Tom went on for six hours. SIX HOURS. We started at three hours, and he extended by three more. I was new then and thought, hoped, our 'date' would somehow crescendo into sex or something a bit more exciting than telly and a bag of chips. It never did and I spent the last few hours counting the taxis driving up and down George Street. At least the room had a view.

Our meetings were usually only ever three hours. Three is what I could handle, three is what I braced myself for; 180 minutes of watching sport, eating Pringles, and listening to unfunny jokes.

One windy Friday night, as the red digit flicked to my final minute, Tom uttered the words that made me freeze. 'Samantha, shall we extend for another hour?'

I felt my blood drain from my cheeks. Poor Tom, I'm sure he'd have seen the dismay written all over my face – if only he would look at it. The extra cash I'd get was tempting, but no. It was past midnight. I was exhausted. I just could not do it. My cheeks ached from smiling, my eyes were fuzzy from the red digits on the clock and the names of half the AFL team in Hawthorn annoyingly taking up far too much space in my head.

I couldn't count another 60 minutes. 'Tom that is so sweet of you, but I will fall asleep and that is not fair to you,' I said gently. Tom, being sweet, understood. 'See you next time,' he said, pecking my cheek. 'I'll bring some cheesy Doritos so you don't get hungry.'

My manager, Raquelle, was an ultra-professional, a fair but firm manageress. She was always impeccably dressed in designer clothes and Chanel shoes, with her streaky hair always pulled back into a tight bun – an instant facelift for someone over 35. 'Next time you don't want to see a client, I'd prefer it if you let me know, Samantha,' she half-scolded. 'I just won't send you to him again. You've just cost us $600 by not extending.'

I wanted to tell her to fuck off. She wasn't the one who had to sit through the bloody AFL for hours and nearly die from boredom. Instead, I said: 'Oh Raquelle, I'm terribly sorry.' I suppose I did feel a bit bad; I had a good work ethic and I didn't like letting her down. And yes, I could see her point. She had been in the business for a long time, and both clients and the girls respected her ethic. Her goal was to make the brothel more money. For me, you cannot put a price on your mental health.

But back to Joe's sugar babies – well, that's a different kettle of fish, clearly. It seems they would do anything for a buck. And now blackmailing? No working girl I know would ever do that.

Joe cheered up when I knelt down and started to massage his balls with my hands, then rubbed his hardening cock against my tits.

'Oh, Samantha,' he groaned, thrusting his hips back and forth, sliding his hardness into my mouth. 'Do you think we could meet outside of here, could you be my sugar baby? No one would know . . .'

I smiled. Poor, dear Joe. Always looking for the next high, always looking for something better and never content with what he had.

'Darling, you couldn't afford me,' I whispered into his ear as I straddled his cock. We both laughed. It's amazing how easily men forget their problems when they have a tight pussy clamped around their dick.

Even if I wanted to see Joe on the side, it's not wise. There is a notice pinned up on the board in the girls' room at The Bordello:

LADIES WILL BE INSTANTLY DISMISSED FOR SEEING CLIENTS PRIVATELY AND STEALING IN ANY CAPACITY, INCLUDING CLIENTS.

Other reasons for getting fired include being pissed while on the job, hustling and overcharging clients, and not using condoms for oral and sexual intercourse. Nor are we allowed to gossip about clients or other girls, and under no circumstances is bitchiness allowed. Ever. 'If we find out girls are being bitchy and spiteful, we will get rid of them instantly. That kind of behaviour is not tolerated here,' said Raquelle. Ha! Don't you wish office bosses were as ethical?

So let's go back to my first-ever client. Like losing your virginity (and wasn't that a wonderful experience for me), fucking your first-ever client is something a sex worker never forgets. I struggle to remember my first client of the day. It doesn't matter how busy my day was, how many penises I had to check, how many sad stories I had to hear or spotty backs I had to massage. When I'm driving home, it's mostly a blur. But my first client, almost two years ago now, will be forever imprinted fondly in my memory.

'Right. Tissues, wipes and plastic bags are in the drawer under the bedside table, and remember to put the towels in the wash afterwards,' said Nina, the madam. I was at an upmarket appointment-only penthouse on the lower north shore, a good place to start my new career. Quiet, friendly and three working girls on the books, including me as of today. 'Rick's in the shower. Don't worry, he's a regular; a lovely man. I see him sometimes in the mall with an Asian woman, a lot younger than him, but of course, I walk straight past him . . .' And her voice trailed off.

'Is he good-looking?' I asked nervously.

'Er, no, darling. The girls and I call him Mr Burns, like from *The Simpsons*. You'll be fine. He knows it's your first time.' And with that, she walked off and shut the bedroom door. I sat perched on the end of the bed in my new expensive black G-string and push-up bra, waiting for Mr Burns to get out of the shower and join me.

Oh my fucking God. Was it too late to get out of here? What was I thinking? I'm a mother for fuck's sake, two years away from 40. I glanced in the mirror. My expensive lingerie seemed alien on me. I was an imposter. Calling the number in the local newspaper had seemed so exciting, so silly, like a dare to myself. Could I really do it? Should I? Would I? Here I was. *Fuck*.

Here in a plush penthouse within a pleasant-looking residential block of units, opposite a church of all bloody places, where I was about to have sex with Mr Burns for a few hundred bucks. There was a concierge downstairs and a decent gym. But in this three-bedroomed apartment there was a whole lot of whoring going on.

I was about to dip my toe in. This was not about money, truly. I wasn't on the breadline. I wasn't being forced to do this. I already had a great job running a busy news desk on a national publication. I was *choosing* to put myself through this.

Was this a test, some kind of reality show I was forcing myself to star in? I am addicted to stories, especially other people's stories – and now I was becoming a story. What was it about? I don't know. I was yet to work that out. But now was not the time.

I scanned the room. The view was top dollar, the Harbour Bridge and Opera House in full view. I looked at the little white boats gliding effortlessly across the harbour and wondered about the people sailing them, probably having a lovely day on the water. If they only knew what was going on in a room not too far from them. I glanced at Rick's clothes, neatly folded on the fabric chair: jeans, a plain black T-shirt and his shoes – white-and-blue runners – tucked underneath. He wore Asics, not Nike. He probably wasn't that cool or intimidating. Was he a bit of a nerd? I hoped so.

He's tidy, I thought. Surely that had to be a good sign. Suddenly, the door opened. In walked a pale, skinny man with a balding head, pointy face and a thin smile, a white towel wrapped around his bean-pole body. Mr Fucking Burns.

'Hello, Samantha,' said Rick, still wet from the shower. He extended a long, skinny hand towards me. 'It's lovely to meet you.'

'Hello, Rick,' I smiled, swallowing my fear. 'Do you know you're my first-ever client?'

'Sh! Don't put that pressure on me!' he laughed. 'You're probably always going to remember me! I'd better be good!'

And just like that, the ice was broken. Rick was human. More than that, he was nice. I liked him. But that didn't mean I wanted to fuck him. Oh my God, I had to take control of this situation. I'd never had sex with anyone I wasn't attracted to. But Rick had paid $380 for this experience. I had to perform. Just pretend to be someone else, I thought. Someone else, somewhere else, in some other place. Let the performance begin, Amanda. It's *showtime.*

I slowly peeled off Rick's towel to reveal his hard, skinny cock.

'Nina told me you were beautiful, and she wasn't wrong,' he murmured, pulling me on top of him, unclipping my bra. He sank his lips onto mine, his tongue exploring mine urgently, passionately, while his fingers slid inside my panties.

'Can I?' he whispered, tugging at them gently. Nodding weakly, I could feel myself get wet as his fingers gently circled my pussy, then moved deeper inside. Was I supposed to be enjoying this? What were the rules? For a moment, I was lost in the passion, the urgency, the naughtiness of it all.

'Put the condom on,' he whispered. 'I need to fuck you.'

Fumbling for my bag, I reached for the condom, tore it open and slid it on his cock. Enjoying this now, I straddled on top of him, sliding up and down on his hardness, moaning quietly. I closed my eyes. I didn't want to see his face, his pointy features, his wrinkles or the sweat building up on his top lip. It wasn't Rick, it was that hot guy in the newsagent's today . . . the one with the big arms . . . oh yes . . . yes . . . *yes!*

'Oh Samantha, I'm sorry but I think I'm going to cum,' he groaned, pulling me closer. And as I felt his cock pulsate inside me, I caught my reflection in the mirror. I saw my spray-tanned legs straddling his and thought about the fact I was having sex for money with Rick, in this strange room, and suddenly, I climaxed. It was a moment I will never forget. Elton John's

'Tiny Dancer' was playing in the background, my body was still shaking, and I was wrapped in the arms of a complete stranger.

Afterwards, there was no awkwardness, no wondering who was going to make the first excuse to leave the room. We still had 20 minutes or so left. We lay in each other's arms, talking, laughing, like a couple.

'So, what was I like?' he asked cheekily.

'Great,' I replied. What else could I say? The sex was good, the situation bizarre, and normally I wouldn't have looked at Rick once, let alone let his fingers dance all over me. But it wasn't awful. I didn't do anything embarrassing. I had managed to give Rick a good time.

Eventually Nina knocked on the door, which meant time was up. Rick grabbed a towel and headed off to the shower, leaving me to quickly tidy up. Condom in the plastic bag, sheets off the bed, heels back on, lingerie back on, just in time for Rick to come back. We pecked on the cheek and Nina saw Rick out.

'Thank God that one's out the way,' I breathed to Nina, flicking on the kettle. 'He was lovely, you were right, Nina –'

'Oh darling, there's no time for tea,' she replied briskly. 'You've got Steven in 15 minutes. Doctor. Married. Bit of a bore. We call him Toad Face. Chop chop, in the shower!'

That day, after Toad Face, came Bad Breath and Nice Asian Dentist, and six hours later and with $800 stuffed in my handbag, I called it a day. I drove home in a daze, my mind racing, every bone aching in my body, and gasping for a drink. It was my first day as a sex worker and I'd survived. Not just that, I'd enjoyed it. I didn't feel raped, abused or degraded. I didn't feel I needed to stand in the shower for hours and scrub my vilified body. I felt euphoric.

34

Samantha

'I bloody did it!' I shrieked to my best friend, Tab, calling her on my way home.

'You are fucking joking,' she replied excitedly. 'What ... what ... what was it like? Oh my God, Amanda, you DID IT! Are you okay? Was it okay?'

'Easier than I expected,' I said, speeding across the Harbour Bridge. But how do you explain the feeling of strange fingers and hands exploring, touching, your body wet with sweat and cum ... how do you explain that it's not just wild sex but also banal and insanely normal conversation, laughter and the odd fart (them not me).

'One client did give me a good recipe for lasagne,' I murmured, flicking my indicator in the direction of the eastern suburbs, back to my beachside home.

'*What?*' Tab asked.

'Sultanas,' I replied. 'The trick is to add a few sultanas.'

AMANDA
Power

How does a nice girl like you end up in a place like this, eh? *Nudge nudge, wink wink.*

As much as I would love to tell you about my ex-husband and my life with him, I won't. He is good man, a fantastic father and a pretty decent ex. And that's all that needs to be said. So there.

Besides, what do you really need to know? My ten-year marriage to him is really nothing to do with what I do now.

He didn't kick me out on the street (in fact, I walked away with a generous settlement). He was neither abusive nor violent (in fact, he was kind and soft). He's not an absent father (he insisted on 50/50 custody). He was a nice husband. He is a nice man. It was me. It was, *truly.*

My fascination with men and sex was born a lot earlier. Remember how I lost my virginity? That was just the beginning, the opening of Pandora's Box.

Amanda

I went to a very nice and conservative school for girls in London. No boys allowed. There was a boys' school up the road, and the highlight of my morning Monday to Friday was putting on my almost white lip gloss and smartly walking to school, and when I saw a boy in red-and-black uniform walking towards me, I would feel that desire again. I was never allowed to talk about having a crush or a boyfriend or anything at all to do with boys and sex in our household. It was not the done thing. As far as my mother and father were concerned, as long as we didn't talk about it, it didn't exist.

Boys and men noticed me. I knew I had some kind of power, that as females, we have power. Once, on the way to school, a car, a black Golf, screeched to a halt. Out jumped a boy in a different coloured uniform. He handed me a note and got back in the car and drove away. 'I see you walk to school every morning. You're beautiful. Call me.'

I called, his name was Russell, and we were heavily petting a few days later in his boyishly untidy room.

Another time, another car screeched to a halt. It was on a weekend, when I was with my sister on the way to the lolly shop. This man ran out, went to buy the nearest bunch of flowers he could, and practically threw them to me with a note with just his name and his number. Funnily enough, another VW Golf, a gold convertible.

This one turned a bit sour, and he started to stalk me. We never had sex, we never even kissed. I didn't even call him. But that bloody gold Golf would follow me. I'd see it parked outside my family home. He even shoved my sister off her push bike because she wouldn't give him our home number (mobiles weren't invented then.) This went on for weeks, months. 'Just leave me ALONE!' I shouted at him once in the street.

'It's because you are a racist!' he spat back. Racist? No, I didn't reject him because he had dark hair, it was because he was weird and I was 14 and I had no idea how to handle the situation. Mum just got angry if I mentioned anything about men or sex; even the conversations disgusted her. So what was the point? It seemed like I had to learn everything myself.

This was another life lesson for me. I realised men could turn nasty if they didn't get what they wanted. I started to dread the flash of gold driving down our street, slowing down at our house.

With hindsight (always a wonderful thing), I can see now that there were plenty of times men took advantage of me. Now it makes me angry, but back then I only felt confused. When I was 16, Steve the builder came to our home to fix something over the space of a week. I can't remember what now. Mum went out to pick up something for dinner, leaving Steve and I alone. He was in his forties, with a glistening bald head and tidy moustache, and I was still a reasonably naive school girl.

But I had been brought up with manners and would always make him a cup of tea with a few chocolate biscuits. One day, as I was making his tea, he started to massage my shoulders. 'Gosh, Amanda, aren't you tense? It feels like you really need a massage. I can feel so many knots here, and here, and here . . .' as his fingers circled down, down, down . . .

I froze. I stared at the kettle, watching his reflection in the hot metal surface. I started to sweat in my red turtleneck. What should I do? Was this something I'd encouraged? It was only tea! Maybe I shouldn't have offered those biscuits, it was my fault, I was too nice . . .

'Um, ah, would, would you like sugar, Steve?' I mumbled, feeling sick in my stomach.

'Come and sit here, Amanda,' he replied, taking my hand and leading me to the kitchen table. 'Just relax.' And he started to massage my back, slowly yet firmly.

'You have such amazing breasts,' he went on. 'You know, my sister is a topless model. Here, let me show you a photo.' He pulled out of his wallet nude photos of a woman. I nodded, in shock. Where the fuck was my mother?

'Oh wow,' I said nervously. 'She looks great.' Was that okay? Not too sexy? How could I make myself look ugly? My mind was racing. Think, Amanda, think. I pursed my lips together thinly, hunched my shoulders over, stuck my belly out. There, was I repulsing him yet?

'You could do this, show your body off,' he purred sickly. 'You could do this . . .'

Blank. And there the memory ends. I am 100 per cent certain nothing happened. I do recall him instructing me not to tell my parents about our interlude. I do recall telling my parents that Steve gave me a massage. And I do recall never seeing Steve again. Nothing was ever said on the matter. But I blamed myself. Steve must have reacted from a signal from me. I believed that. A part of me still does. Despite being a shy teenager, wearing a turtleneck and a daggy corduroy skirt, I blamed myself. I was too nice to him.

But haven't most women experienced an incident like this? Haven't we all been victim to some kind of sexual harassment or abuse? I'm not talking about getting wolf-whistled at by tradies (I've always thought it will be a sad day when they stop whistling at me). I'm talking about the comments at work, the friendly slap on the bum, the talking to your breasts.

Once, while employed in a busy newspaper in London, the top newshound approached me in the local pub. I was flattered. He was smart, good at his job and respected – and he was taking the time to talk to me! In front of everyone! My colleagues nearby and I fell immediately quiet as he approached me. What pearls of wisdom, what advice would he have for me from top dog to young gun? 'So tell me, Amanda,' he snorted loudly at me. 'We've all had a bet in the office that you're wearing these really big *granny knickers*.' A pause while everyone looked at me. Jesus Christ. What the fuck should I say?

'Jeremy,' I whispered in his hairy ear, 'I'm not wearing any knickers.' Silence. Jeremy looked at me, before guffawing into his pint. That's right. I could be one of the boys. He wasn't even the worst. Another time, a good-looking cocky lad asked me the question that had obviously been bothering him since my contract started. 'Amanda, who have you been fucking to get this job?'

'Damian, darling, who *should* I be fucking?' was my response. Ha ha, laugh laugh. Amanda can handle it. (For the record, I fought my way into the media through sheer hard work and determination. Not because I opened my legs.)

Wasn't this the norm in working life? It had been most of mine. At 18 I got my first proper office job, filing, filling out time before going to uni. My boss was a married South African man who was vertically challenged but not bad looking.

I remember him pushing me against a wall by the photocopier as I walked past once. 'See!' he hissed, an angry look in his eyes. 'Look what you do to me!' and he grabbed my hand and made me feel his erection.

'I'm sorry?' I stuttered. Me? I'd done this? I'd somehow caused him discomfort? Was it my fault, was he angry with me? He was my boss – was he going to sack me?

Yet, blindly, I didn't realise that what he was doing was wrong. I accepted his lifts home, the fact he would try to touch me at work, would tell me sorry tales of his unhappy marriage, and I assumed he was flirting with me and liked me. 'When my wife goes away, I will take you to my house and make you a cocktail.'

'Oh that would be lovely, thank you,' I replied. Was that the right answer? Thank God she never went away.

I didn't see it as sexual harassment until decades later. Were all men like him?

It wasn't all bad, though. A well-known man from my local suburb in London, who owned a few high-end shops, and spent summers in the South of France and winters in Aspen, took a shine to me. He wasn't very handsome, but had a nice mop of blond, curly hair and wafted around smelling of money and an exciting life. He never asked me out, never made a move. But the one thing he did say made me beam.

'Amanda, you always remind me of one of those girls in the James Bond movies. You're the sort of girl that will be travelling around in a helicopter one day.'

I don't know why his words stuck, but they did.

Chapter Three

SAMANTHA
A hairy encounter

'I've been waiting an hour and a half to see you,' he said gruffly, standing up, clutching his mobile phone in his hand.

'Oh darling, I'm terribly sorry to hear that. I'll make sure I'll be worth the wait,' I whispered into his ear, taking his hand, leading him up those stairs and into a bedroom, a walk I'd done hundreds of times by now. I'd been at The Bordello for over a year and was doing well. But while I knew my job inside out, clients like this were a little more unusual. No girl likes a difficult client, especially one who's pissed off. And he was big, too – a stocky bald Greek man in his thirties, with veiny muscles straining out of his Nike T-shirt.

'How long would you like to stay?' I asked, inspecting his already hard cock for any signs of an STI.

'Forty-five minutes,' he shot back. 'I haven't had a fuck in three months, so this better be good.'

He handed me $390 – including $50 for kissing – and undressed for a shower while I went to the cashier. 'Forty-five minutes in room 1,' I said, handing her the cash. 'And not one minute more!' I called out to her nervously, walking back towards the room with a bucket full of ice, my evening bag of condoms and lube tucked under my arm.

Just outside the room, I could hear the shower running. I closed my eyes and took a deep breath. I wondered how this was going to pan out. How was I going to handle this one? Here we go, Samantha. Showtime.

I made him a drink and tried to spark up a conversation. 'So, why no sex in three months?'

'It's not easy to meet women on an oil rig,' he replied, with almost a smile on his serious face.

'Oh your poor, poor darling,' I whispered, kneeling in front of him, slipping a condom on. 'Let's see what we can do about that then . . .'

He groaned and grabbed the side of my head with each hand, forcing me onto his hardness, which was already leaking with pre-cum.

'Give me that filthy pussy, you whore,' he grunted, grabbing my hair, tugged at it, while throwing me onto my bed.

For a second, I felt fear. What was he going to do to me?

I soon found out. He flipped me on my stomach, prised open my legs forcefully, and before I could protest, shoved his hard cock into my pussy as far as he could.

Could I protest? Not really. My head was buried in the pillow, his elbows were locked either side of my skull, squashing my ears. Jesus Christ, was he going to kill me?

'Take this, slut,' he said, pounding it in, again and again. 'And this, and this, I want to bruise you, you're a slut, a dirty slut!'

Ouch! Something was hurting. Time out. Time OUT.

'Stop!' I tried to shout, but only came out as a mumble, considering I was face-down in a pillow. 'Stop!'

As quick as a flash, he stopped, flipping me over so he could see my face. 'Are you okay, Sam? I thought you wanted it like that . . . I'm really sorry, Samantha. Shit, are you okay?'

'Rami, it's fine, you were great,' I replied, scratching my head. 'You did everything right. You were just leaning on my hair and it was pulling my extensions out.'

I pulled one long brown rattail-looking extension out of my scalp and hid it before he saw.

'I'm never going to get it right, am I?' he said glumly, lighting up a cigarette.

Ahaha. Got you. You thought I was being abused. 'So much for being in control!' you were probably thinking, half concerned for my well-being, half gleeful at being right about your assumption: that sex in brothels is dangerous.

No. You see, Rami and I have a deal. We've been seeing each other for a few months now, once a week or so. He wants to up the ante on his sex life, to have sex a bit different from his normal routine. His sweet God-fearing girlfriend, he says, likes sex with lights off, nightie pulled up, a packet of wet wipes ready. Rami wants to have rough and dirty sex, but there's no one to have it with. He adores his woman and would never leave her, yet he wants to be satisfied sexually.

I happen to like a bit of rough (though controlled) sex too, but when I ask clients whether they could possibly pull my hair, or give my bottom a playful slap, the majority refuse to because they are heartily against any form of violence – especially against women. The butt-slapping I have had to endure has been pathetic. Slap? Bless them, they wouldn't even kill a mosquito with some of their little taps. Endearing little things.

Rami and I talked briefly about his girlfriend. He would never cheat on her, so visiting me was the only release he could get. 'Have you tried talking to her about sex?' I asked.

'Yes, but she gets angry,' he replied.

In my experience anger is often code for fear. His girlfriend might have been scared of letting go, or not being in control.

I couldn't solve Rami's problems, but I could give him a chance to air his fantasies, to have the sex he always wanted without hurting his girlfriend mentally or physically.

Now, this is important. I am not suggesting that women should do what their men want in bed even if it doesn't feel right for them. For example, I don't do anal sex. I've tried it and I don't like it. It hurts. Unless the client has a penis that would make a button mushroom look frightening, I am comfortable saying no to clients who ask, even *plead* for anal, even if they are prepared to give me an extra $400 for it. Amanda feels the same way. I did it once with a lover in Melbourne, even though it wasn't my idea, and it ripped me apart, quite literally. At the airport the next day, I had to whisper tearfully to the awfully nice but shy-seeming pharmacist that my anal region had a tear and I was going to find it hard to sit down on the flight.

I could have sworn his glasses steamed up. 'Read this,' he whispered back, handing me an information sheet on bottom problems. 'And wipe these on the affected area.' He passed me some antiseptic anal wipes. I even had to rope in my best friend, Tab, to inspect my bottom for damage. (She does really love me.) I won't divulge her comments – even I have dignity – but I made a solemn promise to myself while hovering over my seat on Qantas flight 12 to Sydney. Never ever again is a penis even nudging my nether regions.

I have a funny little saying I like to repeat to my real-life boyfriends if they keep asking for bum sex: 'Not until we're married, darling.' Well, at least I think it's funny. They rarely ask again.

But back to Rami. I don't know what the answer is. I rarely do know. But I've come to learn – painfully – that you can't get everything from one person. His partner may tick all the boxes in loyalty, cooking and cuddling, but when it comes to dirty filthy fucking, that is one box I will happily tick for her. As long as he doesn't rip out my $1200 hair extensions while trying.

Or, more importantly, as long as she doesn't rip them out if she ever finds out.

AMANDA
I heart Sydney

Sydney has been kind to me, kinder than my hometown in grey London ever was. When I signed a two-year contract with a magazine and jetted off to the other side of the world, I knew I wouldn't be back.

'You can kiss your career goodbye,' a reporter snorted at me when I told him I was moving to Sydney. He had a point. We had worked together on one of London's most respected tabloids (if those words could ever belong a sentence together . . .), him in showbiz, me, a junior starting out on the features desk. The editor's budget included money for my friend to have his cocaine nose reconstructed, and for me to go halfway around the country for a story. It was an exciting time in London: the era of phone hacking, The Spice Girls, and Princess Diana. I would chase celebrities down the street for a comment and sit outside pop stars' homes for 12 hours with a photographer in the hope of a getting a naughty snap. In one of my less proud moments, I shoved a Dictaphone in Paula Yates's face and asked her if she was a bad mother, mere weeks before she was found dead from an overdose.

Liam Gallagher from the band Oasis once told me to 'fuck off' and I've got photos of Peter Andre cuddling me at the launch of one of his albums.

My editor one evening informed me that Damon Albarn from the band Blur was going to be at a dog track in London. 'Go there and get a story!' he barked at me. 'And wear something sexy for Christ's sake.' It was 10 pm on a Saturday night.

I was going to a heaving dog track in the east end of London by myself. I sat in the bar and waited, wearing a white clingy dress, heels and too much make-up. It didn't take long. Damon clocked me the minute I walked in. To cut a long story short, we got a taxi to a nightclub together and shared a few drinks while he whinged about his pop-star girlfriend. I got a story, my editor got his headline, and Damon was none the wiser. It was hardly journalism at its finest. But I was young and pretty, and my editors knew how to best use me.

But I wasn't proud of the person I was becoming. I did things I am still ashamed of. I made up quotes, lied to people and once even stole a photograph of a soap star from the very proud owners of an East London Chinese restaurant. I pretended to be a fan of an actor to try to get into his private home. 'Look, just fuck off you little nasty cow,' the woman with him spat at me, trying to close the door while I was prising it open with my foot.

With real-life stories, horrific accidents and grieving families, we were told to get in quick, get the photos and do the interviews while the families were still in shock.

So while you may frown about my job now, I can assure you I have done far, far worse.

I remember being in a trendy shoe shop in Covent Garden when I was about 24. I was trying on a pair of ultra-fashionable – but ugly – shoes. They were horrible; they looked like shoes polio sufferers wore. But everyone was wearing them.

'Should I buy them? What do you think?' I asked the sales assistant.

'I dunno!' he smirked. 'Ain't you got a mind of your own?'

I was shocked into silence. I bought the shoes knowing they didn't look nice and never wore them.

But the sales assistant was absolutely spot on. I don't think I had a mind of my own back then. I went to a posh school where we were told how to act and what to do all day. Then I would go home to a mother who seemed to be in one big bad mood for years, so I'd cower upstairs in my bedroom until told to come down for dinner.

I wasn't allowed phone calls during the week, or to have friends visit. If any of my friends dropped by, Mum would make them feel so uncomfortable by ignoring them or being rude they'd end up leaving. I desperately wanted to grow up quickly so I could leave this place behind.

I was 26 when I moved to Sydney, and while that sounded mature, I had no idea who I was or what I wanted in life. Find a man, get married – isn't that what people did? Marriage, or more accurately, commitment, scared me. I never seemed to get it right with men. I was a late bloomer. Not with sex, but with confidence and self-esteem. I really had no idea what I wanted.

Things seemed a bit happier on the job front. The media in Australia, thankfully, was not as cut-throat as in Britain. In my first week on the job with a magazine in Sydney, my editor pulled me aside. It seemed I had a habit of making people sound better in quotes. 'Amanda,' she said nicely. 'Stop making things up. Here in Australia, we don't alter people's quotes in any way.'

I looked at her incredulously. 'What? You actually write what people say?' I couldn't believe it. How dull!

But I grew to love the conservatism and gentleness of the media. Unless you were a rugby league player or a politician, they pretty much left you alone. The public seemed to be more interested in another speeding camera on the M2, or the price of petrol, not naughty vicars swinging in the suburbs. Leave that to the Brits.

I'd had a few boyfriends in London, but no one serious. Mum wouldn't allow them in the house so relationships and sex were done elsewhere. My friends began to see me as the girl always in a relationship. 'You've never been single for a second!' they'd joke. I needed boyfriends because I needed to escape my home and my mother. They were my ticket to freedom. By the time I was 25, I'd moved out on two different occasions to live with a boyfriend. It wasn't that I adored these men and convinced myself we were to marry. I knew my life with them wasn't forever.

But then, I moved to Australia. And I met curly-haired Christian.

Curly-haired Christian was crazy about me to begin with. He would write me long emails, call up to three times a day to ask me out, and sometimes he'd turn up at my work to drive me home. Christian was the ultimate Sydney party boy, and I was completely enamoured with him. We became quite the item.

Life was good. I was now 29 and features editor on a women's magazine, lived in a trendy one-bedder in a pretty suburb dotted with cafés and parks, and apart from Christian's weekend cocaine habit, we were going great guns.

One summer's day, a few weeks before my 30th, I woke up with a blinding headache. My best friend, Tab, and I had our morning run planned, and I didn't want this headache to get in the way of that. It was still early in the morning when we met up. We jogged around Centennial Park while my head continued to thump painfully.

Our routine was always the same: we'd run, then go home to get ready for work, then Tab would pop up to my unit to pick me up and we would pootle through Darlinghurst to get a coffee, before reluctantly parting ways to go to work. And of course we'd spend the whole day on email to each other. We had a lot to talk about!

And thank God our routine was always the same because if she had not been there early that morning, I might not be here today.

'Tab, I feel really shit,' I said rubbing my head on our way to work. This migraine was a killer, my worst yet. My vision started to go blurry, I couldn't see my shoes or my feet – or in fact anything under my waist. Just blackness. 'I must need a coffee or something.' God, was my caffeine addiction that bad?

We walked the ten or so minutes to Darlinghurst, but it just got worse. I stopped dead in my tracks. I couldn't even cross the road – the cars seemed to be driving in slow motion, people walking past me looked like they were walking in chewing gum, everything looked surreal. I grabbed a lamppost – to hold me up.

'What the fuck . . .' I held onto the post tightly. 'Tab, I can't walk. What's wrong with me?'

We just happened to be outside a café. 'Get me a coffee, quick,' I said weakly. 'My blood sugar must be really low.'

But Tab was worried. 'I'm calling Christian,' she said. 'You're not right.'

I cradled my head-between my legs, but I still noticed a man staring at me from across the café. He had a strange look on his face. Was it concern? Or was he about to come onto me?

For fuck's sake, I can't look good like this, I thought. Can't he just stare at someone else today?

Christian turned up within minutes and held me up as we all walked into the medical centre, which just happened to be across the road.

'I'm Doctor Teenan,' said the man, shaking my hand. I looked up. Him. The man from the café.

'It's you,' I murmured when I recognised him.

'I was looking at you,' he replied, checking my pulse. 'I suspected something might be up but I wasn't sure. Here, sit down, let's find out what's wrong.'

Something was wrong. Something was very, very wrong.

In short, after a CAT scan and more tests, it was apparent I'd suffered some form of stroke. Though it was only minor, I spent one week in the stroke unit of St Vincent's Hospital, just me hanging out with frail pensioners. It was there that I was diagnosed with a hole in my heart.

'There's the bugger,' murmured the cardiologist, peering at my heart on-screen. 'Do you see that black bit there? Your hole is about the size of a 50-cent coin, so yes, quite big.'

Christian was squeezing my hand as I blinked away tears. Jesus Christ, was I about to die?

'It's nothing to worry about. You have a patent foramen ovale,' he explained. 'It's a flap that didn't close over when you were born. About one in five of us have it. Yours just caused a little stroke, that's all.'

That's all? *That's all?*

Having a near-death experience like this was numbing, but that was just the beginning. A few days later, the magazine I worked for folded. Sales weren't great, so management decided to shut up shop. And then I turned 30. So in the space of just over a week, I'd had a stroke, lost my job, and turned over the hill. Hardly cause for a celebration. I had a quiet, awkward dinner in a restaurant with friends but went home and cried afterwards.

Oh, sorry, I forgot. Silly me. It gets better. The day I came out of hospital, numb, bruised, vulnerable, curly-haired Christian dumped me. 'Hey, Amanda,' he said sheepishly, driving me home, not daring to meet his eyes with mine. 'Now you're out of hospital 'n' all, well, um, I'm just a boy that likes a beer and a line of coke, and, well, you can't be in that scene any more with your heart and everything . . .'

Brilliant. I felt totally and utterly alone. My family were on the other side of the world. I assured them I was fine and Mum was quick to believe me. 'Oh darling, if you're sure you're okay. Oh, let's invite that nice doctor to our house in France.' This was my mother's solution to my health issue.

'Sure, I'll mention it to him,' I mumbled. Why don't you come and visit me instead?

I'd just been diagnosed with a fucking great big hole in my heart, I'd lost my job and now the boy I adored no longer wanted me. I think that's when my descent into sadness began. At a loss over how to get over this feeling, I did the only thing that seemed to make sense at the time. I bought a dog. A little Jack Russell–Chihuahua cross called Georgie.

I adored him and he replaced a gaping hole in my life. If only he could have replaced the hole in my heart as well.

A few weeks later, I went back to the cardiologist for a check-up. 'Where's your boyfriend?' he asked, ushering me into his room.

'He dumped me,' I replied quietly, my tears dripping onto my white hospital gown.

The cardiologist looked up at me and I swore the vein on his forehead started pulsating. Was he about to have a heart attack?

'Excuse my language, Amanda,' he said, shaking his head. 'But what a fucking cunt.'

It was the first time I managed to crack a smile in days.

Chapter Four

SAMANTHA
A day in the life of . . .

There were four clients today. One four-hour booking with one of my regulars, a Lebanese man who told me he was a builder, but carries thousands of dollars in cash and bags of cocaine. What did he build: drug empires?

After him was the skinny Indian doctor who pays me an extra $50 to stick my finger up his arse (with a glove on, of course). Does he get jealous when he has to do it to his patients? I always wonder, amusing myself during this awkward procedure. He has a partner but admits he could never ever ask her to do it. Well, I can't see how it would really come up in conversation, can you? Unless you actually uttered the words, 'Can you please stick your finger up my bottom?'. Most people would find it an awkward topic to broach.

Then a nice little surprise for me in the afternoon: a very handsome 22-year-old engineering student who proclaimed his love for me.

After the engineering student I had a polite and good-looking Spanish computer software engineer who lived in New York with his wife. He was visiting Sydney on business. 'Can you pleasshhh dresssh up as skoolgirrrl?' he purred in a sexy Spanish accent. My school days were 20 years ago. How old did he think I was? Thank God for the dim lighting.

Four clients over a ten-hour shift, the total earned: $1900. A good day in my office.

I drove home, had a cup of tea and heated up some lasagne, and watched *Breaking Bad* in bed with my dog, Georgie, for company. I always appreciate my dog after a day's work. He doesn't want anything from me. I can fart, poo or walk around naked, and he doesn't bat an eyelid. He loves me as I am.

I don't often find myself reflecting on the day at work. I barely remember the sex or the conversations. And I certainly don't sit there and question the meaning of life, of the morality of my job. It's a job. Sure it's exciting, it's different, it's naughty. But at the end of the day, it pays my bills and gives me freedom.

Samantha has disappeared for a few days, and Amanda is exactly where she loves to be the most: home.

I love my job, and I love Samantha. She's fun, sexy, womanly and confident. She can be in the middle of her lunch break when a client books her and, within five minutes, go from exchanging vegan recipes with the other girls to whispering sweet and sexy nothings to a nervous science teacher.

The constant performance can be exhausting. It's not just the physical work. Listening to men talk about their problems all day requires emotional energy too. When I am with them I have to be present, focused.

The most gruelling interview I recall as a reporter was with a woman who had been gang-raped by eight men in

Melbourne. I remember her voice changing as she recounted every minute and shocking detail of the ordeal. In particular, I remember the way she talked of the rain pelting down on the bonnet of the car. 'I focused on the rain,' she'd said quietly, her voice changing. 'I couldn't feel the pain. I disconnected. I just felt the rain splashing onto me and onto the car.'

But that's not me. I don't take myself off to some happy place in my head. I don't need to. The experiences aren't bad – they're just draining.

There's a lot of giving involved in my job, and by the end of my shift, I've got nothing left to give.

I fell asleep once, on the shoulder of the world's most boring accountant. He was telling me in great detail about the new person doing the wages in his business – an old people's home. My eyes were heavy, I seriously could not listen to any more of this. That was it. I was gone. One way ticket to the Land of Nod. I even started to dribble on his wrinkly, freckly shoulder.

'Would you like a cheeseburger with that?' I murmured loudly, in my sleep.

'Cheeseburger?' he snapped at me. 'What are you talking about? Were you sleeptalking?'

Shit, Samantha. Get out of this one. *Fast.* The man is not paying $450 an hour for you to fall asleep on him.

'Oh, darling,' I soothed, stroking his cock, soft, smooth and small, as it nestled in my hand like a little dead mouse. 'You just make me feel so relaxed, truly. I must really like you to do that, I would never fall asleep with a client, ever. I see you more like my lover . . .'

As his cock hardened, I breathed a sigh of relief. You've got to love these simple creatures.

AMANDA
Visiting hours

After being dumped, and nursing a holey heart, I moved in with girlfriends in a bright and clattery house in one of Sydney's vibrant suburbs. I was working for another magazine now, as features editor still, and was enjoying being single. I was a little bruised emotionally and probably a bit vulnerable, so when one of my flatmates told me about this lonely old man in the hospital where she worked who lay in his bed waiting for visitors who never turned up, I thought it could give me something rewarding to do.

'I'll go and visit him,' I announced, when she told me.

'Really? He'd love that. Poor thing, always smiling, but he must be so lonely. I never see any family around,' Tania replied.

So that's what I did. A few afternoons a week, I'd walk to the hospital after work, armed with magazines and chocolates.

I'd pull up a plastic chair and spend an hour or so chatting with Ned.

The gratitude was selfishly heartwarming.

'You're a lovely girl,' Ned would say sweetly as I helped him fluff up his pillows, or fetched him a cup of tea. I would ask him about his family, but he would shake his head sadly and change the subject. He must have been at least 80 – I figured his family were probably either dead or didn't give a shit.

Ned would sometimes 'accidentally' flash me. Now, I don't know whether they make old people wear pants or not in hospital, I wasn't sure of the undies rules, but Ned did not wear anything waist-down and he made sure I knew it.

Of course I never said anything. I didn't even look, or at least tried not to. A wrinkly set of balls and a flaccid old man's penis just wasn't my thing.

So I ignored the silly flashing of this senile old sweetheart, and continued to visit him a few times a week for a few months, until one morning, I got a phone call at work.

'Hello, I want to speak with Amanda,' snapped a woman whose voice I didn't recognise.

'Speaking,' I said slowly, trying to think. Shit, had I written a story about her and misquoted her? Or was she a lawyer telling me to expect a letter? It wouldn't be the first time . . .

'I'm Joy, Ned's wife,' she replied briskly. 'And don't tell me you don't know who Ned is.'

Ned? The old man in hospital? 'Yes . . .' I mumbled, not making sense of any of this.

'Keep your hands off my husband!' she suddenly shrilled. 'Don't think I don't know what you're up to. He may be older, but I know what he's like. Has anything happened between you two yet? Tell me the truth. It's the least you can do, chasing after my husband like you've been doing.'

For the first time in my life I was lost for words. I'd been trying to do something good, visiting a poor old man, who I wrongly thought was all alone, and it turned out he had a wife the whole time. But hang on just a minute. I wasn't trying to bloody seduce him – what the fuck had Ned been saying about me? Not only had he been trying to stick his half-dead knob in my face at any given opportunity, but also had a wife and kept it from me. Was he actually deluded enough to think he was in with a chance? It would have been laughable if I wasn't now stuck on the phone to an irate pensioner who was accusing me of moving in on her geriatric husband.

'Look, Joy, I'm a 30-year-old woman. I am not interested in your husband,' I replied, trying to stick up for myself. But it fell on deaf (probably genuinely deaf) ears.

'I know your tricks. Don't you think I don't know your tricks!' she said, her voice getting louder. 'What has he been saying to you? Has he tried and kissed you yet? I know what he's like –'

And suddenly, it clicked. My anger disappeared, replaced by pity. This poor woman must have been living in a constant state of fear that her husband was cheating on her. At her age. *At their stage.* How many years of panic and worry had she had to endure, fretting that Ned was always trying to get it on with anything that moved . . .

'Sorry, Joy, but Ned is how old exactly?' I said, finding my voice and cutting her off.

'He's 79,' she replied tartly.

'And how long have you been married?' I asked.

'Forty-nine years,' she answered, her voice softening.

'And you're telling me that after all those years together, men his age don't change?' I said slowly.

Silence, then a sniffle. 'No, love,' she replied sadly. 'Men don't change. *Ever.*'

Chapter Five

SAMANTHA
Number 43

Here's something interesting. Cocks don't age. Seriously. A few of my clients are over 60, and while their balls droop like dried-up tea bags and their pubes go white and fluffy, their erect penis stands hard and firm without a wrinkle to be seen. Unless these men are having Botox in their one-eyed trouser snakes, I have come to the conclusion that penises do not age. Feel free to discuss amongst yourselves.

Let me tell you about Bob. Bob is 73. He is a dairy farmer from the South Coast of New South Wales, and he looks like one too, with a healthy glow, good strong hands, which are often covered in the odd scratch or cut on his knuckles, and a white beard.

'Hello, Bob,' I smiled warmly, meeting him for the first time in the intro room. Bob had booked me for two hours without meeting me. All he'd seen were my photos, which didn't even include my face.

We made polite chit chat, and then he dropped the clanger. 'Samantha, my dear, I have a disability,' he admitted as we walked up the velvet carpeted stairs towards the private rooms.

I swallowed, trying not to let my fear show. 'That's okay, darling,' I replied. 'What is it, a bad leg? You're hard of hearing?' I desperately hoped to myself that it wouldn't be anything too nasty. I had a particular fear of deformed feet . . .

He shook his head. 'No, darling. I can't seem to get a hard cock.' He spat the word 'cock' out proudly, looking at me teasingly for some kind of reaction.

Bloody hell, I thought. Not only do I have to spend two hours in a room with a man who looks like Father Christmas, but I'm also going to have to work extra hard to get him erect. I wondered if my hourly rate was worth it for this particular job.

'Oh, I'm sure you'll be fine,' I smiled sweetly. 'You're in the best of hands.'

Poor Bob couldn't contain his excitement as I peeled off my dress. 'Oh, Samantha, look at those boobies . . .' and 'Oh, Samantha . . . look what you've done to Mr Smith!'

It was hard not to pat myself on the back – my tricks were working, my *ooohs* and *aaahs* and back arching and lip curling and tongue sticking out was working and Mr Smith, Bob's penis, was hard and stayed hard until a little squirt filled the condom and I could finally, finally take a break. 'Oh thank you Bob, you were fantastic,' I breathed sexily. Hey, what's a little white lie here and there?

'So, Bob, are you married?' I asked nervously – I never know how my clients will take that question.

'Oh, yes. For 45 years, three sons, seven grandchildren,' he replied proudly, his fingers circling my big, brown nipples.

'And is she ... I mean she's here, still alive, you're still married?'

'Oh yes! She is. We have a lovely marriage, but no, she doesn't know I come here.' Bob took a big slug of his whisky and coke and looked at me.

'You really want to know, Samantha, don't you?' he said, his healthy country-aired eyes twinkling. 'You want to know why I come here?'

I nodded, breathing in the suspense. While other girls couldn't give a shit about the clients' lives, I *had* to know. It wasn't so much nosiness, it was a need. I was first and foremost a journalist. My thirst for having to know everything was still there. I was fascinated by my clients, why they were here, whether they were married, what they did for work, how often they came here. It felt like I was living in a reality show, and I was getting addicted to it. While I could act out Samantha, the reporter in me felt like I was privy to a never-ending succession of real-life stories and, to be honest, I found them compelling.

If I get to know my clients, what makes them tick, I can give them exactly what they want. An overworked, stressed bank manager would not want the same service as a horny young surfer dude. A single drug dealer does not want the same service as a married dentist. The more information I have on my clients, the more I can tailor my service, and the more likely they are to return, which means more regulars on my books, and more money.

Bob sat up and fluffed the white pillows behind him, his still semi-erect penis poking at me.

'I got to the age of 65 and I'd never had sex with another woman apart from my wife. Not one. I decided I was going to do it, so I looked up this place, after all, it's supposed to be the best, and made a booking. I'll never forget Sandy, the first girl I had sex with since my wife, Joan, she was a lovely girl from the north of England . . .'

I smiled. 'So coming here was a thing to do on your bucket list?' I replied, stroking his arm.

He chuckled. 'I suppose you could say that, yes.'

'But you're 73 now, Bob. That was eight years ago.'

'Yes, Samantha, I'm addicted to the bloody place now. I've been sneaking to Sydney all this time to come and see you ladies. You're number 43. My special, sexy Samantha is number 43.'

I looked at him, half-shocked, half-amused. 'You've been here 43 times?'

'Oh, yes, and I can name every single one of you ladies. Sandy was one, then Tara, Jenny was number three – didn't think much of her, a sour-faced French girl, Alicia, was four, oh and that lovely Chrissie, the Perth girl, was five . . .'

And on he went.

It was funny, really. Good old number 43. Not a chance of keeping Bob as a regular, then; he'd be on number 99 before the end of the year.

We had sex again, and made some more small talk – Bob telling me about always losing his false teeth (this from the man who could remember the name of all 43 women he'd slept with besides his wife) – until the buzzer went. It had been an entertaining few hours but there was still something niggling me. 'Bob, if I may say so,' I said as he got out of the shower, 'you don't seem to have a problem with getting an erection.'

'I know, darling,' he grinned, throwing his white bath towel on his hard (again) cock and leaning back, showing off his robed manhood. 'I always tell that to the girls so they work harder!'

Nick was a nice man. A bit hopeless at running his glitzy brothel in one of Sydney's affluent suburbs, but I could tell during my interview that he was a decent bloke. By now, the plush three-bedroomed penthouse on the lower north shore where I got my first gig had sadly shut up shop for good, and the other girls and I were out of a job. There was no way I was going back to magazines. Not when I could work the hours and days I wanted for five times the money I'd make in the media. This job wasn't perfect, as I would later find out, but at the time I didn't see anything but the benefits of working in a job as autonomous as this. I was making great money and I was spending more time with my kids.

Why would I want to go back to dating men who weren't up to scratch? I'd only end up feeling used and pissed off. This way, men had to pay for me if they wanted me, and I no longer felt any kind of resentment towards them. I didn't hate men: I loved them.

So I went back to flicking through the internet in search for an upmarket boutique establishment. I called a few agencies, but no one seemed to answer their phones, except one that didn't employ older women.

'We only employ girls under 21,' snipped one woman. More likely they *tell* you they're under 21, you cow, I thought.

Another place, an elite escort agency, was keen. I was offered an interview the next day. Then they found out I had a tattoo.

'Sorry, the clients don't like tattoos,' explained the woman behind the desk.

After a few more phone calls, I found Sex Kittens.

'The thing is, I'm 38,' I explained nervously to the gushy, deep-voiced manager over the phone as I was walking the dogs. 'I look really good, but if you aren't interested in older women, it counts me out.'

'Oh, darling,' she breathed sexily. 'Our clients love older women. So much more experienced. Come and see us today. Are you free now? We'll pay for the taxi.'

Her desperation should have warned me off, but I needed a new job. After a quick shower, I threw on some jeans, a white singlet and tan boots, and off I went.

The décor was pretty nice, if a little tacky. It was a far cry from the penthouse suite, which, though an upmarket hotel room, was a little on the bland side. This was a proper brothel. This was where good money could be made. A huge diamond disco ball glistened over the pool table, and there was a bar that served drinks from Moët to Belvedere vodka.

'Sit down, love, and Nick will come and meet you,' said the honey-voiced manager. She ushered me to the black leather sofas.

Nick was a tall man with long hair and a thin moustache wearing an Adidas tracksuit. His beady eyes nearly popped out of his head when he saw me – I was clearly above average in his books.

'Why do you want to do this work?' he coughed nervously, fingering a clipboard with an official piece of paper, making clearly IMPORTANT notes (probably marking things off like 'great tits, nice legs, posh bird').

'I like money, Nick, and I love sex,' I replied confidently.

Nick looked up immediately. 'Can you start tonight?'

It was my first and last night at Sex Kittens. It was awful. The girls were rude. One, a chubby blonde in a white, stained

Supré dress, insisted on sitting in front of me legs akimbo, displaying her pink fleshy bits and chewing gum loudly, staring at me.

Another woman, obviously the big cheese as she was the only one under a size 14 and didn't have tattoos all over her, kept talking very loudly about how dirty the rooms were, the fleas in the beds and the dried vomit in room 10. (When I confronted the manager about the conditions, she told me it was a ploy by that woman to put me off. It worked.)

The clients were even worse. I saw a man who looked like an Oompa Loompa, a skinny café owner in his fifties who snorted up so much cocaine I thought he was going to have a heart attack, and a 25-year-old who tried to take the condom off when I wasn't looking. It was vile. I felt dirty, not in control, disgusted. The showers were broken, the sheets were dirty. This was my first experience of a brothel and I hated it. There was no training, no advice. 'Just get out there and meet them,' hissed the now-moody manager, practically pushing me out to the meeting rooms. It was not the same as the upmarket North Sydney penthouse. This was degrading. I'm better than this, I thought, zipping up my dress for the final time.

I marched to the front desk and, seething, announced to the manger: 'I'm leaving.'

She looked up from her magazine, shocked. 'You can't . . .' she said, her voice wavering. 'You're on till 4 am.'

'Oh yes I can,' I snapped back. 'I want my money and I am out of here. This place is disgusting. The girls are rude, you're rude, and the clients are repulsive. The rooms are dirty, everything is broken and I refuse to be here a minute longer.'

She tried to argue feebly, but I held out my hand. Reluctantly, she pushed nine hundred-dollar bills into my shaking hand.

I marched out, slammed the door behind and got into my car. Thank fuck. That place made me feel dirty. I pulled down the visor and looked at myself in the mirror. What the fuck was I doing? All dressed up with my now-wonky fake eyelashes, heavy blush and smudged red lips. Not only was I over the hill, but also I was kidding myself. It wasn't empowering, it was awful. Thank Christ I wasn't the type of person to hold on to bad memories. It was over Red Rover and never to be returned to again in my head or in my life. In fact, this whole escorting game was a bloody joke.

That's it, I thought as I screeched down the highway. I am never, *ever*, doing this again. I didn't care about the money or the flexibility. I'd stick with office life, get the bus to work five days a week. I'd find a cheap nanny. Back to normality, that's what I'd do. After all, you can't put a price on mental health . . .

I cheered up when I got home, my safe place, and clicked the kettle on. I could put that horrid place out of my mind – and my body. I didn't want to think about it anymore.

Until I opened my bag. I'd left my fucking wallet at Sex Kittens. The manager had put it in the safe for me. Seriously. Could it get any worse?

It was 3 am. I was in my tracksuit with a cup of tea. I drove all the way back to Sex Kittens – a good half-hour drive – and feebly asked the rude manager if she could very possibly get my wallet out of the safe, hoping that she had completely forgotten my rant at her barely an hour ago.

'Take it,' she spat, practically throwing it at me. So what did I do? I did the thing women so often do when they feel guilty – I overcompensated.

'Look, I'm really sorry about earlier and of course, I would love to work here next week,' I said, feeling a ridiculous mix of guilt and relief that she actually gave me back my purse. 'Really, maybe if I did days rather than nights . . .'

'Oh great!' she exclaimed, brightening up. 'You're probably more suited to the daytime.'

She scribbled my name onto the roster for Monday, Tuesday and Wednesday, 10 am–5 pm. 'Wonderful. We'll see you then.'

I knew two things as I gently closed the door of Sex Kittens behind me. 1) I was never going to set foot in that place ever again. 2) I had a commodity and I was going to sell it. I wasn't any old sex worker. I was high class. I was going to find the best and work there. Fuck normality.

AMANDA
The Bordello

I'd heard of The Bordello years ago. I'd read in the papers that the controversial and colourful owner had put in development plans to open the country's biggest and best brothel in the city, and there was a lot of hoo-ha from the residents about not wanting a knocking shop on their street, thank you very much, complaining it would cause noise and more crime. The irony was, with a security guard patrolling the establishment and nearby streets every night from six in the evening till seven the next morning, you probably couldn't live in a safer street.

The clients mostly drove here and parked underground, or taxis would do a quick drop-off. And the girls didn't hang around on street corners, we hurried in quickly, wearing big sunnies and baseball caps to avoid being seen.

I knew it was *the* place to work, that the girls were high-end and beautiful, the clients rich and famous, and that I could make a lot of money. I'd seen the girls on the website – they looked like they had jumped out from the wrinkly arms of Hugh Hefner.

After my stints in the penthouse and then Sex Kittens, I finally felt brave enough to give The Bordello a call. I knew that an educated, well-travelled, classy woman who looked not-bad in the right light was in demand in these places. Young wasn't always an advantage in this game. Maturity and good conversation often stood head and shoulders over great tits. Both was a bonus.

Nick from Sex Kittens was still trying to woo me back with ridiculous offers and Nina, my very first madam, kept texting me to tell me a few of my old clients were asking where I was working now.

I knew I was good enough for The Bordello. I was ready. I scanned the website. It looked intriguing – there was a gym on the premises for the girls and a solarium (neither of which I've ever seen being used, incidentally), and the rooms looked sensational. Two levels, with the second level reserved for clients staying three hours or more.

I was still working in magazines, but only part-time. My interview in Australia's best brothel would be during my lunch break – the only time they could fit me in. 'Just popping to the city to get my eyelashes done,' I whispered to the PA. It wasn't going to arouse suspicion: I was working in the beauty department now. Long lashes were not just part of the job, they were a requirement.

Of course, what I was dying to say was: 'I'm just going to a brothel for an interview! Can you believe it? Me! Do you even know what The Bordello is? You stay here and pretend to look busy – I'm off on an adventure! Toodle pip!'

'No worries. See you soon, Amanda,' smiled the PA, her eyes flicking to her watch.

Jesus Christ. Was she really going to time me? I hated corporate life and with my dalliances into the free and flexible sex industry, I was losing my patience with it.

My stomach churned as I hailed a taxi. I wasn't going to any old establishment. I was going to the best. I had every right to be nervous. I couldn't fuck this up. A quick spray of YSL and a slick of Dior gloss, and of course, trying to explain where I needed to go to a confused cab driver who of course had no idea where he was going. 'Is it a one-way street?' he asked, punching the name of the street in the GPS.

'Look, do you know The Bordello?' I said eventually. Fuck it, why should I care what he thinks? I'll never meet him again. 'Can you just drop me off outside the front door?'

He glanced at me through the rear-view mirror and raised an eyebrow.

'The Bordello?' he said, in a thick accent. 'You want to have sex with someone?'

'No, I'm going for a job interview,' I replied, staring straight back at him.

'It's a very good place, always busy, but very expensive,' he smiled, shaking his head. 'Beautiful ladies. They will love you.' And with that, he turned round and gave me a leering smile, showing his tobacco-stained teeth. 'Here's my card, miss, call me and I will come and pick you up . . .'

Instead of snapping at him to hurry up, I smiled sweetly and thanked him. Rudeness wouldn't have got me anywhere.

We eventually pulled up outside an unassuming grey building. If you didn't know it was a brothel, you could walk right past without even noticing it.

Clutching my mobile, I rang the doorbell. I glanced up. A security camera was pointing straight at me. I smiled – I knew my interview had already started.

The big grey door clicked open and I suddenly felt like Dorothy in *The Wizard of Oz*, as she finally gets to see behind the curtain and meet the Wizard. Except that unlike Dorothy, I wasn't disappointed.

'Hi, welcome to The Bordello!' smiled a tiny well-dressed blonde, holding out her hand. 'I'm Roxy, I'm the daytime manager here. Come through to the office and we can have a chat.'

We made eye contact and shook hands. I liked her. Roxy was probably in her late twenties, attractive, no make-up except maybe for a touch of foundation. Her uniform was black pants and a stripy shirt, with kitten heels. I glanced down. Chanel. Wow.

Out of the corner of my eyes I could see a water feature and a big red armchair. And it was hard not to notice the grand staircase in red velvet carpet that led up to the boudoirs. I could hear laughs and the sound of phones ringing, cool, unobtrusive music playing from speakers. Once again I was struck by how amazing this place was inside, such a stark contrast from its outside – a grey, windowless building.

The office was not a typical-looking office. It was a room for girls and their clients. There was a bed (I rather think all offices should have one!) 'for our disabled clients', Roxy told me later. 'Because it's the only bedroom downstairs, we can cater for wheelchairs.'

At one end of the room was a minibar, and at the other, a queen-sized bed with a separate bathroom. All marble, all glistening.

We chatted, mostly about what I wanted from this job (flexibility and great clients) and what hours I preferred. 'I won't lie,' said Roxy. 'You're definitely a day girl, more for our corporate clients, the businessmen. What size bust did you say you had again? And how old are you?'

I paused. 'Do you want me to be honest?'

'Of course,' she smiled, looking up.

'I'm 38.' There goes my job . . .

'Okay, lovely, we'll just say 30,' she murmured, scribbling more notes. 'And when can you start?'

'Next week?'

'Great.' She smiled, looking up, a twinkle in her eyes. 'I think you'll do very well here. Welcome to the family.' She shook my hand firmly and showed me out.

She said yes! I was going to be a Bordello girl! This was so exciting.

Tab was happy for me, but concerned too. 'Should you be doing this? Is it safe?' Her worry angered me. What did she know? Tab, in her cosy comfortable life with her husband, watching reality shows and Instagramming her lattes, knew nothing of this world. She had no idea about the prestige of being a Bordello girl. 'I turn lots of girls down,' Roxy had told me in the interview. 'Only a select few meet our standards.' See – I was lucky to get through. And as for the safety, well, that question made me smile. Was it less safe than the real world? Was it safer than picking up a random guy in a bar, when you're both drunk? Don't more wives get bashed by their husbands every night in the 'safety' of their own home? Men paid a lot of money to come here and they weren't going to waste their time and money being an arsehole. We had buzzers if we needed them. We had to use condoms for oral sex *and* penetrative sex.

Tell me, how many times have you slipped a condom on a man you met in a bar before you gave him a blow job? Do you always use condoms during sex? Of course not. I have had more scary moments with men in the real world than as an escort. I've put myself in more dangerous situations as Amanda than I have as Samantha. The only danger I was in was falling asleep in the arms of a rambling accountant. Sex at The Bordello could not have been safer.

Tab had my back, but she had no idea, no understanding of how impressive this job title was to working girls. If you were going to work in the sex industry, you wanted to work at The Bordello. *Everyone* knew that.

I knew I could take leave whenever I wanted. I knew I could work one day a week if I wanted. I knew I would be making good money.

I felt more excited then, than at any other job offer I'd got. Roxy didn't know my real name or where I lived. And she didn't care. All she knew was what I looked like. She didn't care what my degree was in, nor did she try to woo me with promotions. All I had to do was turn up for my allotted shifts, be a good worker and not steal clients, and I'd make lots of money. 'Our best girls can take home over $2000 cash a shift,' Roxy said. I nodded, a surge of determination taking over. What did it take to be one of their best girls? I was going to figure it out, and I was going to do it.

Chapter Six

SAMANTHA

My tribe

So what does one wear to one's first shift as a high-end escort at The Bordello? A very expensive and fitted dress from Wheels & Dolls Baby, of course.

'I need a dress to wear to my first shift at The Bordello,' I confessed to the peroxide blonde at the counter dressed in retro clothes.

'This,' she said, not even raising her pierced brow, as she shoved a clingy leopard print mini-dress at me. 'All the Bordello girls love this.'

As I twirled in the mirror, to the admiration of the sales assistant, I felt proud butterflies. 'The Bordello girls.' I loved the way those words sounded. Did I finally belong somewhere?

I looked good and I knew it. I was slim and fit, having worked with a personal trainer a few times a week, and had a large bust. I was no stranger to a few jabs here and there, and my role as a beauty editor had served me well: I knew all the right make-up tricks, such as applying bronzer to highlight the contours of my face (God knows how many times I'd written that sentence in an article). But in the end I learnt far more useful beauty tricks from other working girls than from my years in the beauty world. For example, did you know talcum powder is a cheap alternative to dry shampoo? Olive oil works wonders as a make-up remover. Never brush your teeth before a booking: it opens your enamel to infection. Some of the girls even washed their you-know-what with Listerine but I would NEVER recommend that.

And one rule that every woman knows, sex worker or not, is that too much make-up is very, very ageing. And the men aren't a huge fan of it anyway. I lost count the number of clients that asked me to not wear perfume (they didn't want to go home smelling of YSL), or would it be okay if I wiped my lipstick off.

As time went by, I got to know the other Bordello girls and they were ordinary, normal, pleasant women. There were no supermodels (just fantastic airbrushing on the website), no stuck-up bitches (they wouldn't last) and no addicts (except sex addicts, maybe). The girls worked a variety of 'day jobs', from lawyer, nurse or counsellor, to HR manager, student or even forensic detective. Their ages ranged from 19 to late forties. I didn't just feel part of this secretive gang, but also that we were from the same tribe. These were my people, and we had some stuff in common: we could disconnect emotionally from sex (it was after all just sex), we'd got sick of doing it for free and we liked making good cash. Some of the girls had boyfriends, husbands, ex-husbands, girlfriends, while others like me were single and preferred it that way. Some had told their partners, friends and family what they did, while others kept their business private. Some preferred to keep to themselves at work, and we respected that, but there were always cackles of laughter emanating from the girls' dressing room; always a sense of sisterhood, camaraderie. I'd seen most of them naked, faked 'lesbian sex' with a fair few, and shared many, many laughs.

We would give each other advice on anything, such as how to deal with a huge cock (we never liked those), threesome lesbian bookings (that's a secret), as well as what to do in five-hour party bookings (which means pretending to do cocaine when you don't do drugs). The thing about Bordello girls was that we were smart enough to know that once you got wasted, a few drinks here, a few lines there, on repeat five times a week, you lost control and bang, there goes your empowerment. You had to keep your wits about you. Smart sex workers stay sober. Smart sex workers stay in control. Smart sex workers have boundaries. And smart sex workers save their money.

Looks-wise, The Bordello catered for every man's taste. Girl-next-door, fake chesty blondes, redheads, skinny girls, voluptuous girls, white, black, Japanese, Chinese, Thai, Indian, Fijian, Kiwi, American, English, South American, French, Italian, Czech, Russian ... we had something for everyone. My confidence improved. I learned to love my body as it was. You didn't have to be thin, just healthy. In fact, I'd been turned down by a client once because I was too skinny, having lost too much weight at that time. And you didn't have to be beautiful; you just needed to have something about you. Men in the intro room would notice a girl from her smile and her eyes before noticing her body. 'It was your energy,' a few did admit to me. Probably bullshit, but I appreciated that line.

The men were just as varied. Mostly nervous, in awe of the glamorous women and the dark, velvety, decadent interior. They didn't feel like princes; we treated them like kings.

Despite this, I was nerve-wracked right before my first client at The Bordello. Shitting bricks. Imagine doing a live TV interview – naked. Colin was pretty run-of-the-mill, mid-thirties, married, pale skin, dark hair and a bit tubby. 'You're my first client here,' I smiled shyly.

His response was a grunt. Shit. It wasn't just ice I had to try to break, it was the bloody Antarctic.

He booked me for an hour sometime in the afternoon. 'On me lunch break,' went another grunt. He worked in the car industry. He emptied a whisky and coke in two gulps, and smoked a cigarette quickly. He fucked me missionary with his gold chain dangling in my face and when he came silently, a few minutes later, his face turned, his eyes went squinty and a bead of his sweat dripped onto my chest.

'Right. I'll have a shower, I think,' he puffed, wiping his dripping cock and stuffing the tissues in the plastic zip-lock bag provided. He showered in silence while I quickly made myself a vodka shot. I said no drinking on the job but I needed something to stem my nerves. 'I might leave now,' was another grunt, as he tied up the shoelaces of his Brookes trainers.

'Sure, but I think you still have time left. I can give you a massage. Or maybe another drink?' God, this was awful. Was *I* awful? This man seemingly couldn't wait to get away from me. Maybe I wasn't a Bordello girl after all. Maybe I was kidding myself. Shit, what if he complained?

'Here,' was his final grunt as he took a $20 note out and left it on the drinks table. 'Buy yourself a drink.'

I sat awkwardly on the bed, not sure what to do. I didn't

want his sympathy tip. I felt obliged to take it, but I didn't like this feeling. What was it – confusion? Guilt? Worry? Yes, that was it – I was worried I hadn't done my job properly. I was paranoid now that I was not worth $450 an hour and Colin had just worked it out. I was a fraud. You know that sinking feeling you get when you realise you've done something wrong at work? That you could get into trouble? That was the feeling I had. But something wasn't right with Colin. His silence was unnerving. What the fuck had I done wrong?

You know by now I like a chat, and usually can talk the most silent of people round to a confession, or at least a laugh, but Colin was a steel trap. I only knew he was married because he wore a ring. If I asked him a question, he would grunt or just nod. Was I such a bad root he wanted his money back? Did I fart without realising it? No man would pay $450 for a fart. Actually, come to think of it, some depraved pervert would – the smellier the better too, probably.

I didn't mention anything to Roxy. Whenever I caught her looking at me that day, I averted her gaze nervously. She was probably trying to think of a nice way to say, 'You're a dud root,' without hurting my feelings.

The next few clients were fine, thank God, easy.

Colin came back months later. To see me. I was firmly established at The Bordello now and had my regular clients. This tubby, sweaty man was smiling at me, reaching out for my hand. 'Weren't you my first-ever client?' I asked, as we walked up the stairs together. Colin was the last person I expected to come back. I'd been so green back then, so new and nervous. He nodded eagerly, his eyes dancing as he stared at my breasts pressing out of my white dress, then down to my pussy. Could he tell I wasn't wearing panties?

'I thought you were wonderful and I haven't been back since to The Bordello because you were never rostered on when I could come,' he murmured, as I unzipped his fly to release his bulging penis. 'I only wanted to come back to see you. I thought of you and your fantastic tits for months afterwards. You gave me the time of my life.'

As he slid his stiff cock into my wetness, I couldn't help but look at my reflection at the mirrored ceiling and smile. You can never read a man's mind. Even a so-called expert like me can sometimes get it wrong. And as I watched his pasty white back heaving back and forth like a sailing ship crossing dangerous seas, that gold chain dangling in my face again, I made a mental note to myself. This is a take-home tip, too. When men are quiet, it's not always about you. Let them retreat into their emotional man cave without pestering them to tell you what's wrong. And maybe, like Colin, nothing is wrong.

Just like the first time, Colin finished, got up, had a shower and left early, pretty much in silence again. But this time, I knew he left a happy man. Colin was obviously someone who kept his cards close to his chest and was a creature of habit. As women we spent too much time analysing what could be wrong, what he could be thinking, what he could be doing, what we could be doing wrong. Relax. I've said it before and I'll say it again: men are simple creatures. Don't overanalyse them. Don't waste your time trying to get inside their head, because no matter how well you know them, or think you know them, you will never, ever get it right. Sometimes men's simplicity is too complex for us.

AMANDA

The beginning,
the middle and the end

I met Luke. We had two beautiful kids. We separated – amicably.

That's all that needs to be said.

Now back to the sex!

Chapter Seven

SAMANTHA
Hungry for love

We all have a low point of our career. Maybe your day at work ended up in a row with a colleague. Maybe you got last month's figures wrong. It happens. You go home, have a glass of wine and unwind. Maybe you chat to a friend about it, have a good cry.

I wouldn't call Melvin a bad day at work. He wasn't rude, nasty or mean. He didn't degrade me, nor did he use or exploit me. I left the room feeling fine. Melvin was, well, I suppose to put it bluntly, dear Melvin was just a bit gross.

It started as a phone call on my day off. I was on my way to have my eyebrows waxed. Blocked number – had to be The Bordello.

'Yes?' I said, hitting the green button on my flashing phone.

It was Raquelle. 'Ah, Samantha,' she said. 'I'm sorry to disturb you on your day off. Is the coast clear to talk?'

I love the secrecy of this job sometimes. I resisted the urge to reply, 'Alpha delta roger positive,' or hum the James Bond theme tune, and instead said, 'Sure.'

'A *lovely* gentleman, a regular, would like to see you. He is flying from Melbourne on business and would like to book you for five hours next week, on Thursday night. Are you available?'

Five hours? That was over $1500 cash. If on the rare chance I had actually planned something to do, I was damn well going to cancel it.

'Absolutely,' I replied, grinning. It was hard not to be flattered.

Thursday came. I drove into work happy and excited. I was about to spend five hours with a powerful, smart, probably handsome businessman. He was from Melbourne for a start, and weren't those men always so well dressed and stylish?

I chose a classy dress – black, clingy and long. Fishnet stockings and expensive suspenders. A quick spray of scent, this time Chanel. Some NARS bronzer, MAC blush, and a slick of nude gloss, and Samantha was good to go.

'Melvin is in room A when you're ready,' the receptionist said. Was that a smirk on her face?

I whirled into the room, my eyes full of hope, expectation and desire. And there, perched on the velvet sofa, clutching a ripped white plastic bag, was Melvin. A short, white-haired Indian man wearing a white shirt with yellow patches under his arms and nylon-looking pants. He jumped to his feet as soon as he saw me, emitting a strange grunting sound.

'Oh, Samantha,' he exclaimed, extending his skinny arms. 'You are so beautiful, so beautiful. Oh, what a lucky man I am, Samantha.' And then he snorted.

Now when I said 'snorted' I mean literally snorted. Melvin had a rather unfortunate habit of making a snorting noise through his nostrils, guttural, choky and kind of gross.

Of course, the professional Samantha was delighted to see Melvin. I gave him a 'loving' kiss on the lips and I linked my arm through his. Five hours. Five very long hours. I stared at the receptionist as we walked past. She winked at me, grinning. Fucking cow.

'Oh, darling,' I replied, trying not to let the disappointment reflect from my eyes. 'I've been so excited to see you too.'

Snort.

Snort.

Snort, snort, snort.

Jesus Christ, I thought, trying not to wince with each noise. How the fuck am I going to do five hours in one room with this little congested piglet?

One thing this job has taught me is that no matter what someone looks like, no matter how fat, bony, balding, spotty or physically impaired they are, if they are a decent human being, they will have one nice thing about them. Whether it's their hands, their feet, their smell, or their voice – I can pretty much find one nice thing about everyone, as challenging as that can be sometimes. And I will focus on it. With Melvin, it was his kindness.

'Samantha,' he said, handing me his plastic bag. 'This is for you. I bought you a present to say thank you for seeing me. You are so beautiful, I am such a lucky man.'

Inside his little ripped plastic bag was a bottle of rosé and something that made me smile – a lot. A box of my favourite chocolates, Ferrero Rocher.

'Oh, Melvin!' I squealed, genuinely touched. 'That is so

lovely. Thank you. No one here has ever bought me a gift before, thank you.'

Glowing, I stored the chocolates on the table by the minibar and opened the wine. I'd look forward to those with a nice cup of tea when I go home tonight. What a kind man. Could I overlook the noise from his nostrils? The constant belching? Could I overlook his tight pot belly and skinny legs? Of course I could. *Think of the chocolates.*

We took our clothes off and drank the bottle and talked, mostly about Melvin. Suddenly mid-sentence he lurched at me, eyes closed, mouth shut, lips protruding, a bit like a bullfrog. My instinct was to recoil but instead I swallowed, took a deep breath, squeezed my eyes shut and kissed him back, lips firmly shut, too. *Think of the chocolates.*

He squeezed my tits and slobbered all over them and instead of the usual quick fuck I had got so used to in these appointments, Melvin leapt up and said in a voice dripping with phlegm: 'I'm hungry, Samantha. Let's get a pizza. Meat feast, please, a large one.'

Up until now I had never seen a client request food but I suppose there was a first time for everything. And it was good news – it meant I could waste a good hour or so faffing around with the consumption of this pizza, or at least, waiting for Melvin to consume the pizza.

I buzzed through to reception and asked them to order a meat feast takeaway. 'Of course, Samantha,' was the reply. 'We'll leave it at the door.' They didn't sound shocked. Melvin was a regular, after all. Maybe they were used to it.

I'm not really a fan of pizza, and wasn't particularly looking forward to eating the meat feast, which to me meant uniden-tified bits of animal entrails scattered all over the dough.

Melvin attacked his pizza like a wild pig, including the same sound effects. I sat on the bed naked, a white paper napkin on my lap and a plate with a soggy slice, staring at him incredulously. How the hell did he manage to stay married with habits like this? He had the culinary manners only a mother could love. I was drifting, taking myself off to some happy vacant place in my head, because my reality right now was a little, um, uncomfortable.

And then something happened that unfortunately brought me straight back to the present time before you could say 'Domino's'. Melvin took a big bite of his slice and turned to face me. 'Samanatha,' he mumbled, while chewing. 'Can I kiss your breasts?'

Before I had time to even THINK OF THE CHOCOLATES, Melvin was on all fours, licking and kissing my nipples, while still masticating on a mouthful of meat feast. I could even feel the warmth of the cheesy topping on my nipple.

But it got worse. Far, far worse. Through his grunting, a piece of ham fell out of his mouth onto my thigh. I looked down in absolute horror at the pink blobby square on my skin. Another slobber, and a wet chunk of beef (or was it bacon?) dropped onto my belly button. Melvin looked up at me grinning, his mouth covered in saliva and globules of soggy dough.

This was awful. I was no fan of food in bed, but when there was a skinny snorting Indian sucking my nipples and bits of pizza dropping from his dribbly mouth onto my body, it became truly, utterly, hideous.

'That feels so nice,' I lied, trying to yank his head up in mock passion, hopefully hiding my annoyance. 'But my breasts are so sensitive. Why don't we finish dinner and . . .'

'You're right, Samantha, dinner is over!' he announced. I felt my muscles relax. Thank Christ. Melvin was beginning to repulse me but it was over now. I could move on. Besides, he was so kind. I had to remind myself of those chocolates!

I flicked the remains of some crumbs away from my stomach and legs while Melvin got up. I naively assumed he would go straight to the shower to wash the meaty smell off himself. But that was wishful thinking. Instead, he jumped up and marched excitedly over to my chocolates. *MY CHOC-OLATES!* I watched him tear open the packet. 'And now for dessert!'

I felt helpless and horrified as he grabbed one of *my* Ferrero Rochers, ripped away the gold paper, and popped it into his mouth. I could not believe what I was witnessing. How rude! You can't give someone a box of chocolates and then proceed to eat them!

Melvin had a strange look in his eyes as he swirled the nutty ball in his mouth. At least he seemed to be chewing it. 'And now for my pretty Samantha's dessert!' He strode towards me, grinning, with chocolate dripping out of his mouth.

I found myself edging further away on my bed until my head was pressed up against the wall and there was nowhere for me to go. Surely no, he wouldn't, he couldn't . . .

He did. Melvin buried his head between my legs. I felt a warm trickling sensation of thick sweet-smelling chocolate being smeared all over and inside me. And not just the chocolate, either. I could feel little bobbles of nuts being pushed inside me by his slobbery, over-excited tongue.

I lay back, my mouth open in disgusted shock. I looked up at the mirrored ceiling, where I could see Melvin's head bobbing up and down, and brown smears all over the sheets (what would the cleaners think?), listening to his grunts. It was like I was being eaten alive by a warthog. As I watched this horror scene, it became quite apparent that this was the lowest point of my career as Samantha.

Later that night, I stood in my shower at home for a good half an hour. The dried chocolate washed away a treat, but those bloody nuts took ages to leave my body completely. I kept finding the odd one in my knickers for days afterwards.

Melvin turned up again a few months later, carrying another bag, this time with the words KFC written on it. His eyes lit up when I walked into the pungent room that stank of fried chicken. My eyes on the other hand wanted to cry.

'I was a bit hungry, Samantha,' he dribbled gleefully at me, shoving the bag under my nose. 'So I've bought us some delicious chicken nuggets . . . they're still warm and crispy –'

'No Melvin,' I said firmly, cutting him off. 'Those chicken nuggets are not going anywhere near me. Do you understand?'

'Oh Samantha!' he snorted happily, ignoring me. 'Wait till you see what I have got you for dessert!'

AMANDA
Freedom

When you've had your kids and been through the merry dance of divorce, being single is a whole lot different from when you were in your twenties, BC (Before Children). It's a damn lot more fun. There's no panic about meeting Mr Right (whom we all know doesn't really exist), no desperate longing to have that baby (been there, done that, got the T-shirt covered in puke to prove it) and chances are you're probably a bit more financially secure, so you can buy your own drinks and take yourself off on your own holidays. The beauty of being single post break-up is that, really, it's just a sex thing.

When Luke and I split, I went on a bit of a rampage. I suddenly had this newfound freedom I hadn't felt in ten years. I had every other week to myself – no kids, no husband, no dinner to make every night, no lunch boxes to fill, no shirts to iron. I didn't even have to do any washing if I didn't feel like it. But back to the sex.

It was a bit like not eating chocolate for a year and then receiving a box of Favourites. You have the green light to gorge yourself.

There was a sexy Spanish waiter, only 27, whom I had a short fling with. Although he was a good few centimetres shorter than me in height, he made up for it in other places. His mistake was buying my kids a goldfish at Christmas. Any man who thinks that a mother with two kids might need another responsibility has no idea about women, no matter how big his cock is. Next!

After him came the hot American soldier whom I met while walking my dogs. It was his last night in Australia before returning to Iraq, and I felt it my duty to thank him for his dedication to serving his country and the world. The way he said, 'Thank you, Ma'am' in a sexy, deep voice after I sucked his perfect Yankee doodle, gave me ridiculous butterflies.

Another young man I 'dated' thought it might be cute to serenade me outside my house at 2 am with a guitar and sweet ramblings. I told him to fuck off and he responded by not only sticking his business card under my door (he was a banker) but coming back the next night and doing the whole bloody song again.

There was the restaurateur who took me back to his place and simply pulled his pants down (I said no politely). Oh yes, and the Swedish 25-year-old who looked like a superhero, who told me he had never fucked a mummy (and then proceeded to send me text messages starting 'Dear Mummy').

A builder working next door would leave me little notes under my door and a tin of chicken soup when I was sick. I arrived at my car one day to find a lovely note stuck on my windscreen, with the words 'You made my day' scribbled on. It was truly flattering.

I had my fun, then I ditched them all. I wasn't looking to buy; I was just browsing.

But it wasn't all shits and giggles. There was the married man who forgot to tell me he was married until we'd slept together. 'I didn't think it mattered,' he'd said earnestly. There was the criminal who was wanted by police (I had no idea who he was until I looked him up on Google). I was stalked by a businessman who, after I dumped him, thought it was socially acceptable to turn up at my house at 4 am, hissing, 'Shut up and let me in.' In fact, his behaviour became so worrying that I threatened to report him to the police and promptly adopted another dog – a big one.

So while I was kicking off toy boys who were clambering at my ankles, the ones I did like were all either unavailable or complete arseholes.

After the initial euphoria of being free and single wore off, I decided: no more. I was going to give myself a break and leave that weird species called men alone. And what happens when you make a decision like that? You meet someone, of course. That man was called Matthew.

Matthew was an older man, a very powerful and rich businessman. He was handsome in a European way. He wore navy Italian loafers and a Ralph Lauren shirt tucked into chinos. His cufflinks were personalised and he looked like he belonged on the streets of Paris or Milan, drinking espressos and reading foreign newspapers.

Matthew also had that one thing that most successful rich older men have: a wife and family. I knew this when I met him, and he never denied it. So when he leant in to kiss me the night we met, I pushed him away, slapped his face and said, 'How disgusting.' At least, I like to think that's what I'd have done. Instead, I pulled him in closer, felt his soft lips touch mine and, when he dared to slide his tongue inside my mouth, I took it invitingly.

We stopped at a kiss that night and I didn't think I'd hear from Matthew again. But he was relentless in his pursuit. For weeks afterwards, I was receiving text messages at all hours. *I can't stop thinking about you Amanda* and *I would like to take you on holiday* and *I could fall in love with you.*

He called me once from his beachside mansion, whispering that his wife was on the sofa watching TV. 'I am so bored,' he hissed. 'I just want to be in your arms.'

When he had to go to London for business, he called me from the aeroplane before take-off to tell me how much he missed me and was falling in love, and as the plane took off on the way home, he called me to tell me he had bought a gift for me. We spoke until I could hear the plane's engines roar.

I started to let my guard down. Ever since curly-haired Christian, I'd been uptight with men. Cold and in control. No one had a chance of getting through to my holey heart. But Matthew? I knew he was wrong on so many levels. But this was different, what we had. The intimacy; the pining.

What have u done to me Amanda? I have never felt like this before.

Jesus Christ, Matthew was in love with me. Obsessed. And I fell for it. I actually believed him. I didn't think about his wife – wasn't that his problem? *I have feelings for you too*, I'd punch out over text. While I was at work I daydreamed of us sunbathing at a fancy resort that he had promised to take me on. Of hot, steamy sex in the hotel room.

Matthew, Matthew, Matthew. I felt twinges of jealousy whenever his wife was calling out to him and he had to hang up abruptly. Stupid woman – didn't she realise their marriage was broken? I know, I should have known better. But I was still able to justify myself. Matthew pursued *me*. He almost made it his career to get me. And boy was he good. I was got.

Romantically enough, all of this wooing and courting was done via technology (even the awkwardly erotic phone sex we had). We had shared only one kiss – a single, simple kiss.

I'm coming to Sydney for business, the words flashed via SMS one evening. *And I'm booking a hotel. I would love you to stay.*

Well of course I'd stay! I was his mistress! They say men never leave their wives, but with Matthew I wasn't so sure. He seemed so obsessed with me. And there were exceptions to the rule, weren't there? Some men did leave, but I could make Matthew very happy.

I turned up at his hotel, nervous yet excited. I wore a cream mini-dress, clingy in all the right places. I turned heads in the hotel bar but the head I wanted to turn most of all was facing the other direction.

'Matthew,' I greeted him nervously, tapping his arm.

'Ah, Amanda,' he smiled, his eyes meeting mine, before slowly moving to my cleavage. 'Please, sit down.'

We drank white wine and talked to the tinkle of a piano being played in the background. It all felt like it was going well until he asked me, 'What are you hoping to get from this, Amanda?'

I didn't really understand – what did he mean? '*This?*' Silly Matthew; so used to talking in corporate-speak, not used to real life, women. We weren't doing business. We were falling in love. Weren't we?

Matthew seemed a bit nervous, almost distant, sitting in front of me with his legs crossed, but I knew it was because of his desire to make a good impression on me. There was a lull in conversation. He swirled his ice in his vodka, took one large gulp, and turned to face me.

'Well, shall we go to my hotel room? I'm rather tired,' he said, stifling a yawn.

I looked at him. It wasn't even 9 pm. A horrible feeling rose from deep inside me, but I squashed it back down. Sex was all he wanted? Of course not. Poor thing must have been out of practice. After all, he probably hadn't been with any other woman besides his wife. Most likely he was just scared of his feelings and the intensity of our love.

'But Matthew, you said dinner, and ...' I stuttered. I'd bought this dress especially for the occasion. I was determined to at least show it – and my handsome European lover – off.

'Oh, okay. You're hungry, are you? Waiter, do you have any bar snacks?' he said, clicking his fingers at the young boy with a wonky bow tie.

'I thought we could actually go out for dinner, maybe near my house?' I said quietly. But I was getting annoyed now. I didn't want a fucking olive. I wanted to be romanced.

'Okaaaaaaaay,' he drawled, looking at me, then his watch. 'Let's go for dinner.'

Dinner turned out to be a sloppy cold pizza in an inner-city late-night pizzeria. 'I don't want anything,' he said, dismissing the menu. 'You eat, then we can go.'

The romantic part was his launching himself at me in the back of the taxi on the way to my house. And I should have known then. But I was so desperate to have this exciting older lover at my fingertips, so excited about this man who had invested so much of his valuable time in me that I didn't really see the situation for what is was. Maybe I simply didn't want to. Once we made love, he wouldn't be able to get enough of me. He'd keep me up all night and I'd probably have to kick him out in the morning . . .

The sex was quick. He was frantic to get inside me, and as soon I could feel his cock pulsate and his body shudder, he pulled away.

'Amanda, that was great. Thank you,' he said, tying up the condom and placing it neatly on my bedside table. 'But I really must go now. I have to get back to the hotel. See you!' He gave me a peck on the cheek, and hopped out of my bed, leaving me naked, my pussy unsatisfied, and still wet, and that feeling I'd squashed earlier erupting from the pit of my stomach. I had a name for it now: anger.

'You WHAT?' I said, raising my voice. 'You've had sex with me and now you're LEAVING?'

But I was talking to no one. All I could hear was his hurried footsteps thumping down my stairs and the harsh slam of my front door. The fucking bastard had just cum and run.

Shaking, I scooped up my mobile and called him. No answer. I pressed redial.

'Amanda,' he whispered, eventually picking up. 'I'm in the taxi –'

'You fucking bastard!' I yelled at him. 'You've completely used me! You pursued me – stalked me even – and now you got what you wanted, you've fucked off. I am furious with you!'

Silence. For a split second I thought he had hung up on me. Then he spoke.

'I am sorry you feel that way, Amanda,' he said calmly, in his professionally measured voice. 'I like you enormously. I just can't do this to my wife. I'm sorry. Goodbye.' Then I heard the loneliest sound in the world: *click. Brrrr.*

I did what people only ever do in the movies and threw my phone so hard against the wall that it cracked. Then I buried my head in the pillow that still smelt of expensive married man and sobbed until my nose blocked up and I couldn't breathe. Didn't the stupid, selfish man realise that she would be far more upset and feel more deceived at all the time he'd invested in another woman, the emotional disloyalty, more than the penis-in-vagina act? Which, incidentally, was over before it barely began. But I wasn't only angry at Matthew – I was so disappointed in myself. How the fuck had I let that happen? How could I not see that happen? I was 37, smart, and I could handle men. How did I let my guard down?

I was alone again.

Matthew rang again a few days later, cheery and blasé, as though nothing had ever happened. It's an amazing gift to have, isn't it? Classic selective memory loss. A gift some men seem to have been born with.

'Look, I just called to say you're a wonderful woman, Amanda,' he said. 'No hard feelings?'

There was no point trying to fight with him. He didn't care. He had a wife. He had a life. He was a powerful man and I didn't really want him as an enemy.

'Yeah, well, you made me feel like a prostitute, Matthew,' I mumbled, my eyes once again stinging. 'I just forgot to charge you, that's all.' I was still raw from his cold and calculated treatment of the incident. I was worth more than that. Far more.

His reply, shall we say, was unpredictable. 'Well, you would make a very good prostitute,' he laughed.

I angrily pressed the red button and thought about what he'd just said. Should I have been insulted? I wasn't. It was the most intelligent thing that imbecile had ever said to me. And even today, I want to thank him for that. Because you know what? He was right.

I made a solemn promise to myself. After Matthew, no man was ever, ever going to treat me like that again. No man was ever going to chew me up and spit me out like that. I'd had jack shit of being used by men. I needed to get control back over them and myself. I didn't feel empowered, I felt manipulated. I'd been through a divorce. I'd already had a few bad experiences with men (who hasn't?). Now I had yet another experience that left a bad taste in my mouth.

Sure, I deserved it; he was married. I should have seen it coming. But as worldly as I was, I was also naive. I didn't have much emotional support growing up, no one to teach me about men or the dating game. I was used to learning things for myself along the way. I learnt I was pretty bad at it.

But Matthew, I have to thank you for being a prick. You and a few others out there have helped me do something that I never would have done without your behaviour. Something didn't die in me after being used like that; something, or rather, someone was born. And her name was Samantha.

Chapter Eight

SAMANTHA
Three's the magic number

It all started off as a normal Saturday shift; I was running late, as usual. 'Afternoon ladies!' I said cheerily to the receptionists as I breezed in through the front door. 'I'll be ready in a –'

'Ah, Samantha, don't go yet,' said Roxy, grabbing the diary. 'I took a booking for you. It's at 9 tonight. You do couples, don't you?'

Roxy gave me one of her pleading looks while chewing the end of the pen.

I looked at her, dread slowly seeping up from the pit of my stomach. I knew this day would come eventually, and here it was. This sunny Saturday afternoon, sometime in November, was the day. How was I going to handle it, I wasn't sure yet.

'Couples? Er, no. I've never done a couple,' I replied slowly, putting my bag down, knowing this was not going to be a quick conversation.

'Oh, you don't? Shit,' she replied, tapping her pencil on the scrawled notes of today's page in the diary. 'Really, Sammy? You've been here a year and you've never done a couple? Hmmmm. I could have sworn you'd done couples. Thing is, Samantha, I told this woman you were our couples goddess and she's made a booking for her and her husband tonight at 9 for an hour. I said you were fantastic. She's so excited. They've never done it before. I mean, I can ring them and cancel if you like. Shame, though, it's $800 an hour for couples . . .'

Oh. My. God. Couples goddess?

She had to be having a laugh at my expense. Talk about throwing me into the lion's den. Actually, make that lioness's den. Men are easy. Flash a bit of boob, twiddle your twat, tell him he is amazing, and it's game over. But a woman? Oh no. You can't pull the wool over a woman's eyes. You can't put on some show for a woman. You can't fake an orgasm with a woman. They're too smart. There's going to be no bullshit, no pretend lesbian kissing. No licking the inside of her thigh instead of her clit. Oh no, siree. She'd be onto me. With women, it has to be all real. Samantha is seductive and fun, she oozes sex. But she's not a lesbian. She's not even bi.

'Thing is, Roxy, I haven't actually seen a couple before so I don't really know what to do.'

'Oh, you'll be sooo fine!' she exclaimed, playfully slapping my arm. 'Seriously, couples are so easy. Half the work! Just ask the other girls.' And with that, she walked off, leaving me standing there with my hand on my hip, wondering how the fuck I was going to get out of this. Or – how drunk I could get before the booking. One of the two.

What kind of weird couple goes to a brothel? What kind of woman wants to see her husband fucking another woman?

They had to be pretty odd. Probably in the swinging scene, I thought, reluctantly opening my locker and pulling out a few dresses for my shift. Tattoos and piercings, drugs and whisky. Why the fuck did I come into work today? My day was ruined.

Maybe the wife would think better of it and back out. Yes, she'd have all day to think about it, realise it would be a huge mistake to throw her husband into the arms of another woman, and cancel.

I couldn't concentrate on anything apart from that looming time – 9 pm. 'You seem a bit distant today, darling,' said Tony, a regular, as he poured me a drink. Tony was a lovely man, in his fifties, a divorcee. He was an expat living in Asia, and was the CEO of a big firm. I loved his stories about Japanese society and culture, of how proud the people were. He told me once he had to make the executive decision to cancel mufti day in his firm, as he discovered the Japanese employees were leaving for the office in the morning dressed in their suits and getting changed in their own clothes in the toilets at work. 'They didn't want to leave their villages in their own clothes on a work day as they didn't want people to think they had been fired,' he told me, his twinkly eyes smiling at me. I could listen to him for hours – and usually did.

I watched Tony as he clinked a few ice cubes into my glass. Sweet Tony. But he didn't need to hear my stuff. The men don't really like to hear that you are with other clients. They know that you are, but they don't want to be reminded of it. They like to think they have a little ownership on you and that to you, they are the special ones, your favourite.

One of my good friends – her working name was Suzi and she was a Spanish dancer from Madrid – had a regular by the name of Curt. Curt was quite an unattractive man who liked having his gnarly, twisted feet rubbed and massaged. Once, when Suzi was off work, he booked me instead, but I had to endure his guilt for our two hours and it was painful.

'Don't tell Suzi I came to see you,' he kept saying.

'Of course not, Curt,' I replied for the tenth time, rolling my eyes behind his back while squirting yet more Sorbelene onto his deformed feet. 'It's our little secret.'

'She'll be upset. I know my Suzi, she's my girl,' he went on, tutting and shaking his head, as if berating himself for coming in when Suzi wasn't on the roster. Curt was a smart man, a big powerful broker with two grown up sons. He was 60-something with gross, knobbly feet. Did he really think Suzi would care? Were all men that deluded?

Of course I told Suzi. 'You're welcome to him, Sam!' she giggled. And we had a laugh. Silly fools that men are – they can't even be faithful in a brothel!

Tony handed me my drink. 'Oh, I'm fine,' I replied, 'Sorry, Tony, it's just, um, work stuff.' I couldn't get the looming threesome out of my head.

'You're leaving?' he shot back, concerned for a second.

'No! No. Don't worry about it,' I smiled, reaching my arms out towards him. 'Give me one of your big cuddles instead.' That cuddle lasted one second and the sex lasted probably four minutes, but come on, you've got to admit, he was easy. Most men were easily pleased. How the hell was I going to please a woman?

The clock was ticking over: 6 pm, 7 pm, and still no cancellation call. The couple was definitely coming.

Back in the changing room, I threw couples into the conversation. I may as well have exploded a tank of laughing gas. 'Seriously, girls,' I pleaded over the cackling. 'I need to know your tricks. Has anyone here seen a couple? What's the secret?'

'Oh they're so easy, babe!' assured Candi, a buxom peroxide from Manchester. Covered in tattoos, and with a heart almost as big as her double Es, Candi had been a worker for most of her young life, first in the UK and now in Oz. The first time we clicked was months earlier, when she grabbed me by the toilets.

'Quick,' she hissed, shoving her iPhone in my face. 'I need you to pose with me for my boyfriend in England. I've told him I'm visiting my auntie in New York and he's getting a bit suss. Could you pose with me for a photo? Try and look like an auntie.'

So not only did I have to pretend to look auntie-like (I presume that meant tits away, T-shirt on) for the camera, but she threw me the phone afterwards to talk to the poor guy. 'What's your real name for Christ's sake?' I whispered to her, covering the phone with my hand.

'Oh hi honey, Michelle has told me *so much* about you.' I put on my best American twang and tried hard not to laugh as Candi nervously hovered around, biting her nails. 'Sure, I'm with Michelle, sure we're having kwoffee. Yep, it's pretty cold up here this time of year.'

It was absolutely hilarious. Of course, Candi got away with it. The poor sod believed her and me. Or maybe he just wanted to.

What Candi maybe lacked in honesty, she made up for in experience. 'With couples, there is one golden rule,' she said, rubbing in her foundation and looking at me through the mirror. 'The only one person who matters in the room is the chick. She's going to be feeling really nervous and really unsure of herself, so it's your job to make her feel like a million dollars. Do that right and you'll be fine, trust me. It's easy.'

Easy. So everyone kept telling me. But if that was true, why did more than half the other girls refuse to see couples? Why did they make gagging sounds and shake their heads? One even looked at me and said: 'Oh Sammy, come and see me straight away after. I could do with a laugh!' 'The girl is a worker almost every time!' one yelled out. Yes, did you know that? Neither did I. Some men bring working girls from other agencies in for a threesome. I'd met a few of these couples in the intro room. The men were always sleazy and the women looked either incredibly bored or super confident.

And, of course, you'd get the complete arseholes with their partners who really did not want to be there. I remember once a husband-and-wife couple who picked another girl I knew, Albany, a striking raven-haired Kiwi. The wife, Albany told me later, was petrified and reluctant, the husband cocky and drooling. They'd had some fun, the woman played along for her husband's sake, then just as she was taking a shower afterwards, relieved the whole thing was over and she could take her husband home safely, he'd called out to her: 'You go downstairs and wait for me love, I'm going to be another hour with Albany here . . .'

'What a prick, right?' Albany had said. 'Her face fell when he said that to her. I snapped at him to be nicer to his wife, and if he wanted to see me, to come back another time when she wasn't there. Then I kicked him out.'

So, you see, some of us sex workers do have codes of ethics. When women's husbands and partners come in to see us and tell us all their secrets and sob stories about empty and sexless marriages over an erotic massage, we do, deep down, secretly think that they're all a little bit selfish and should be massaging their wives instead. I know I do. Sure, women have an equal part to play in their sex lives, and I believe as women, we need to lift the game in the bedroom. But some men really ought to be spending their money on their families and not on me.

I was moments away from getting it on with a woman for the first time in my life. I had to prepare. I changed my dress three times and I wore a bit less make-up. I didn't skimp on the perfume, though. I made sure I smelt nice with Bobbi Brown's Beach.

'Samantha, your couple has arrived. They're in room B,' smiled Roxy, winking at me. 'Don't worry – they look normal. I think. Take them up to level two, and bring a bottle of champagne for them.'

Okay, here it goes Samantha, showtime. Put on your best performance. At least if all else failed I could just get pissed instead.

Keith and Ann were very normal. Married for 17 years, from the western suburbs. They were lovely. I could have kissed them both when their nervous eyes lit up as I walked into the room. In fact, I think I did.

I'm not going to go into too much detail as Keith and Ann probably wouldn't like that, but I will say that Candi's advice was spot on. Ann, a mum of five, felt insecure about her body and wouldn't take her towel off until I told her how beautiful she was and what an amazing woman she was for coming in here with her husband. Her gratitude was warming.

'And you!' I said to Keith, as I undressed him slowly, my eyes still on Ann. 'You are one lucky husband for having such a wonderful, sexy wife.'

'I know. I'm the luckiest man alive,' he said, staring at Ann adoringly, barely noticing I was there. It was, if anything, refreshing.

It was Keith's birthday and he'd had no idea he was being treated to me until an hour earlier, when Ann handed him a gift voucher she had designed herself with my photo on it, accompanied by the caption: 'An hour with Samantha and your wife', and the loveliest message, 'Thank you for loving me so much and making me feel like the only girl in the world xx'.

They marvelled at how posh the room was. 'Just like a fancy hotel, isn't it love?' Ann said, her eyes widening as I showed her around.

'Free drinks? Really?' exclaimed Keith, as I handed him a flute of ice-cold champagne. 'Wow, we weren't expecting that, were we?'

Ann, still timid, looked at my body as I started to undress. 'If only I looked like you!' she breathed as I slid off my stockings.

'Hey, you know this lighting is ultra-flattering, don't you?' I replied. I told her my real age, that I was divorced, had kids, and that outside here, I was really just another normal person. I wanted her to relax, to make her feel at ease. And humanising me seemed to do the trick.

'We've never done this before and we're not sure what to do,' Ann said cautiously, looking at me shyly.

'Let me take control,' I replied and beckoned them to the bed. The next bit is private. While I don't mind telling you about my male clients, who mostly all knew about this book, and like I've said earlier, wanted a starring role, I respect this couple's privacy. What they had together was something special, something sacred, and I will not cheapen it.

But what I will tell you is that they talked about how much they loved each other, how great their sex life was, and Keith whispered to me that he had never, ever been with another woman and was finding this all a bit hard.

It was the most touching thing, and while I did my best at being the goddess, I couldn't help feel I was intruding on this beautiful couple.

'I love you, baby,' Keith kept saying, holding his wife's face close to him.

'I love you too, darling,' Ann replied, and they spent most of the time making love on the bed, while I sat perched on the corner, watching them, with my glass of bubbles for company. And as I watched them kissing, a feeling came over me, one that I'd been beginning to feel more and more often: loneliness. For a split-second it was Amanda sitting there, alone again. Why couldn't I find what this couple had?

All I was used to hearing in these rooms was how unhappy men's marriages were and how it wasn't working for them. This couple taught me that there were good marriages out there; they can work. But it takes exactly that: work. Not all men are pigs. The love that radiated from our room that night glowed inside me for days afterwards. I had been lucky enough to witness it. The trust Ann held in Keith was enormous and I respected her for that. How many women would beckon another woman into the arms of their husband? I admired Ann for her inner confidence and the security she must have felt to let another woman into their marriage. She was busy with children and full-time work, yet her marriage seemed to me one of the healthiest I had seen in a long time.

And I admired Keith for not going gaga when I took my clothes off, for not pawing all over me but instead concentrating on his wife, focusing on her needs and her wellbeing. I was really the third wheel, the outsider. And that was just fine with me.

It ended just as sweetly as it began. Ann lit up a cigarette and grinned at me in postcoital bliss. 'Jeez, Samantha, that was bloody awesome,' she smiled as her cheeks flushed. 'Can't wait to tell the girls at my Monday morning coffee group at Macca's!'

AMANDA
Finding heaven

They say most women fantasise about becoming an escort at least once in their lives. In fact, most women I tell about my job, whether they are housewives, mums, young, old, professional, married, divorced or single, nearly 80 per cent of them, have confessed to me that trying sex work was something that had crossed their mind at least once in their lives. Why they hadn't done it, they told me, was fear. The worry that men wouldn't find them attractive enough, that their weight wasn't 'right' for it or that they would end up dead in a suitcase.

When women find out about my job, they are shocked and curious, but most of all, absolutely fascinated. What are the men like? What is the sex like? How much money do you make?

To be terribly honest, selling sex was something I had thought about for a long time, long before I got married.

My introduction to sex, on that beach in Italy when I was 15, led to my perception: it was dirty and it was all about the man.

Over the course of my adolescence, I learnt that a) men found me attractive and b) I enjoyed having that power. I often found myself in dangerous situations – being drunk with men I didn't know, refusing to go home with my friends and instead staying in a club with a stranger. If there was a dodgy or inappropriate situation to get oneself into, chances are it would be me in it. 'Amanda, your stories are hilarious!' friends would squeal. I was always the one men were chasing, I gained attention wherever I went and had a reputation as the wild girl. My vice wasn't drugs, cigarettes or booze. Give me a green tea over grog any day, a gym membership instead of a lifetime supply of cocaine. No, my vice was legal. I loved, and still love, men.

Every summer as a teenager, my family and I would spend eight blissful weeks in Nice, the city of palm trees, gentle waves lapping onto the stony beach and bustling crowds of camera-clicking tourists. One thing this French resort was famous for was its prostitutes or, as my mother called them, the 'ladies of the night'.

It sounded so glamorous, so exciting. I would watch these women for hours from our balcony. They would stand on the side of the street, with their hand on their hip, smoking long cigarettes, moving only to bend down to cars that slowed down. They would stick their heads in the driver's seat, have a quick conversation with the male driver and more than not, jump in the car, only to return half an hour later to the same spot with their hair slightly out of place and their skirts riding up their arses.

What amazed me was not the whole idea of prostitution, nor the fact that these women were mostly unattractive. There was one woman who didn't even have front teeth (funnily enough, she was the popular one). But the cars that stopped there were always BMWs, Mercedes, even a Rolls Royce. I didn't so much wonder about the women; it was the men I was fascinated by. These men were probably married – some even had baby seats in the back of their cars – definitely rich and could have had any woman they wanted. Why pick up a woman on the side of the street when there were glamourous models in bars and clubs just metres away? But I had no one to discuss this with, no one to explain to me about men or sex or desire or selling sex. It was just me, a teenager, mulling these things over in my head. Men were beginning to play a part in my life; the Italian boy who took my virginity and his cousin who was watching; the sleazy builder and the stalkers. What was it all about? What about nice relationships? Boyfriend and girlfriend? Some of my friends were having sex, on the pill (having been taken to the doctor by their mum), and sex was okay, it was normal, it was allowed.

Sex was forbidden in my family, as an activity but also as a subject. Was that why I was so fascinated with it?

Back home I started to scour the back pages of local newspapers and pore over the adverts of massage parlours, brothels and escort agencies. I was fascinated by this mysterious world. What kind of women worked there? What kind of men visited?

As a journalist, I once spent a night backstage at a strip club. I was dazzled by the shiny lights, the glamorous girls with their layers of pink blush and their skinny legs; I was intimidated by their confidence. 'Here, put a dress on, go out there!' offered a tall Russian girl. She handed me a see-through dress and tried to push me out on stage. I declined politely but every bone in my body screamed yes! I was overwhelmed with curiosity, but scared too. What exactly was I afraid of, though? Rejection?

But I was a reporter; sensible, professional. I wasn't one of *those* girls. I was educated, posh. These girls were probably dumb. They were all junkies. Weren't they? My life hadn't turned out so badly that I needed to dance and strip my way through life. Isn't that what we think? It's because they can't do anything else, right? The fact was that they were normal women, maybe not that different from you: students, single mums, some even married. They chose to strip for a chance to earn great cash in a way that kept them financially independent. Why do we find that hard to understand? Do we think they're going to steal our men, our sexiness? How can we ever compete with women like that?

One day, not long after I'd had my stroke and curly-haired Christian dumped me, I was feeling lonely. Flicking through the pages of the local newspaper, something grabbed me. Da Vinci Girls! Big Bucks Paid! High Class Escort Agency Looking For Girls. Training Given.

Sure, my parents were wealthy, but I wasn't spoilt. While they helped out occasionally, it was me paying the bills, and with a career that was more glamorous than lucrative, it wasn't always easy. Was it time? I could give them a call, there was no harm in that. After all, as a journalist, I'd always be looking for the next challenge, the next story. This would be a great one . . .

I called the number. 'Sure, come in for a chat,' said a friendly female voice. 'We'll give you the address on the day of your interview.' It was of course, like everything in the sex industry, top secret.

I was petrified. I changed my outfit three times that day, and in the end opted for a black-and-white stripy tight number. Once my hair had been blow-dried and my make-up professionally applied, I had quick shot of vodka before I dialled the number.

The voice on the phone gave me the exact address and the instruction: 'Ask for Nikki.'

Nikki looked no more than 19 and was wearing black jeans and a black shirt. 'Hi,' she said, her eyes flicking up and down my body. 'Sit down here and Mick will come out.'

Da Vinci's was a three-room suite on the top level of a block of units. One room was an office, the other was a waiting room with girls lounging around eating Macca's and wearing ugg boots, and the third room was the one I was waiting in. The phone was ringing constantly, with a harassed-looking woman answering one line, putting them on hold, then answering another call.

I sat nervously, crossing and uncrossing my legs.

'Ah, Amanda, hello,' smiled a grey-haired man with a round face, as he came over to shake my hand. He gave me the once-over and pulled out his pen.

'So why do you want to work at Da Vinci's?'

'Um, I need the money? And I like having sex.' Was that the right answer?

'Have you ever worked?'

'No.'

'Good, good,' he murmured. 'Well, let me tell you a bit about Da Vinci's. We are an elite agency. We only have the best clients: celebrities, bankers and so on. You will go on nice trips. You will be treated like a queen. You will make lots of money. But we have one rule here at Da Vinci's.'

He paused for effect.

'Never, ever, fall in love with a client.'

Fall in love? He was joking, wasn't he? I was more worried about not wanting to touch them, let alone fall in love with them. 'Right,' I said slowly. 'And you have to have sex with these men?'

He looked up and laughed. 'The sex is the easy part! Try talking to them!'

Mick liked me. I could tell. Maybe it was my posh accent or the fact that I was a bit older. Maybe I looked more professional. 'You'll do well here,' he said, his eyes flicking over my body once more. 'But tell me. Why does an intelligent girl like you want to do a job like this?'

For once, I was speechless. I looked at him blankly. If this was a trick question, I needed the answer. He was right. Why exactly do I want to do a job like this?

'I don't know,' I answered matter-of-factly. 'I just think I can.'

Was that the truth? I'm not sure. I thought about his question that night. Maybe I was just curious. I'd always wanted to peek behind the scenes and now I'd had my first glimpse. But it was only a fraction of this world. How did it feel to get paid to have sex?

I never got to find out. My parents sent me some unexpected money. I'd managed to save a bit and I was doing better financially. When Nikki called me to ask when I was coming in, I brushed her off with a vague excuse about changing my mind. Hell, of course there was no way I could be an escort, no way I could have sex with a man I wasn't attracted to. But it was there, in the back of my mind. That escort agency was my back-up plan.

I never had a moral issue with it. It was more the safety side of things and, well, my mental health. I loved men and I didn't want to hate them. Nor did I want to hate myself. But the ethics of prostitution? When you have two consenting adults – what really is the big deal? Who would I be harming?

Not everybody I met was okay with prostitution. I had the misfortune of meeting someone like this, some years later, one afternoon after work. I was a writer at the time, married to Luke, and was outside a posh house in a residential street close to the Harbour Bridge, waiting for my lift to arrive.

Suddenly, a Lexus with a red-haired woman driving screeched to a halt in front of me. She got out of the car and slammed the door angrily. And as she came marching towards me, it dawned on me rather quickly that the focus of her fury was me.

'One of those fucking hookers from next door, are you?' she screamed at me, with absolute hate in her eyes. For a second, I looked behind me. Surely she wasn't talking to me.

'I'm sorry?' I whispered, half-petrified, half-confused, looking for the other person she must have been speaking to.

'You heard me. I know what you get up to in there,' she spat and pointed to the house I was standing in front of.

Apparently, I had decided to stand in front of a brothel and she was the unfortunate woman who lived next door. But instead of laughing it off and explaining to her that she had made some foolish mistake, I started to feel fury inside me too.

'How *dare* you,' I said, my voice rising sharply. 'How *dare* you say that to me? I'm a writer. I'm waiting for my friend to pick me up. But so what if I was a prostitute? I would still be a person with feelings, wouldn't I?'

Once she realised that she had just accused an innocent

passer-by of being a prostitute, the woman's face turned ashen. She looked as though she wanted the earth to swallow her up.

She mumbled something about always wanting to be a writer and how lovely my outfit was, and where did I get my shoes?

'Oh, fuck off,' I replied, and clicked off in my heels, texting my friend to pick me up on the other corner. When he finally arrived, and I recounted the whole story in dramatic detail, he laughed hysterically.

'You, a hooker?!' he chortled, giving me a sideways glance as he drove. 'Button was unbuttoned a bit low was it, you old tart?'

It was funny, I suppose. But I felt indignant too. Why should being a sex worker mean a woman would deserve that barrage of abuse? They sell sex, but they're still women: mums; daughters; sisters. Who deserves to be spoken to like that?

And far more importantly, how interesting that such a lovely home with white plantation shutters and a fragrant frangipani tree outside its front door could be a brothel. The allure of the sex industry was still there, tapping gently on my shoulder, teasing me. And while it was just a thought buried deep in the back of my mind, it was still a thought. It wasn't going anywhere.

Chapter Nine

SAMANTHA
Only the lonely

I saw a lot of loneliness in The Bordello, in the men who came in and the women who worked there. Imagine being a spy and not being able to tell anyone what you did for a living? Apart from M, who else did James Bond have to talk to after a hard day in the office?

I was a bit different from the other girls at work, in that I told people what I did. Don't get me wrong, I didn't announce it to the world, or drop it into casual conversation with strangers: 'A latte please, and oh, I'm a hooker by the way.'

I'm talking about boyfriends (yes I had those in the real world) and close friends, a select handful of people in my life. I sort of became a sex therapist for my friends. 'My husband has an enormous penis,' confided a friend once. 'I just don't know what to do with it. You'd know, what with your job. What do you think?'

Or this, from a male friend: 'Er, look Lah-nie, I'm a bit embarrassed telling you this, but I feel I can talk to you seeing as you'd know, but me and the missus haven't had a root in eight years . . .'

Yep, true story. (He wanted advice, not sex, by the way!)

Only one husband tried to crack onto me. *You offer mates rates don't you, Lah-nie?* he joked once over a text message.

Yes, darling. Double for you, I replied briskly. I think he got the message. While I am happy to fuck strangers for money, even I have rules. No people I know. No husbands of friends. Absolutely not.

I tried to keep my life a secret at first. But that was hard for me. And more to the point, why lie if I didn't feel I was doing anything wrong? I saw the mental torture the girls who had secret lives were going through. The angst, the guilt. So many lies to remember! It wasn't the job that messed with your head, it was the deceit that came with it. But that wasn't going to be me. I was pushing 40, a grown woman. I just couldn't see what the big fuss was about. It was just sex.

My friends who knew and loved me only wanted the best for me. They were more concerned for my safety and happiness than passing some kind of misguided moral judgement. What people said behind my back, well, that was out of my control. Don't they say that what other people say about you behind your back is none of your business? But even though I felt comfortable confiding in friends, most of my colleagues didn't. And that, I saw, was a lonely life for them, lying to their friends and their boyfriends.

'I'm only 26,' Sophie, a raven-haired Greek girl from the northern beaches explained to me. 'I haven't got to the marriage and kids bit yet. I've got that all to come. If I tell people what I do, it will stick like mud for the rest of my life. I just can't take that risk.'

I knew my time as a working girl was limited. And I wanted it to be. Or at least that's what I told myself. It was never going to be forever. 'Always have an exit plan,' Nina, my first madam, had once told me. I assumed an exit plan would come up along the way . . . I was only doing this long enough to get it out of my system. I'd make some money, have more time with the kids when they were young, and then hang up the suspenders.

The job was also a chance for a little fun, a bit of escapism. I could leave motherhood at the door, and pretend to be this wildly exciting nymphomaniac for eight or so hours, five days a fortnight. It was showtime and I loved the performance. And besides, I'd created Samantha and she could do whatever she liked.

I could act my way into making money, listening to men and their problems while having nice physical contact. I was lucky enough to be privy to real and honest conversations with men. Was sex therapy only learnt by exams and sitting through uni lectures? Mine was experience-based. I was becoming a full-fledged sex therapist; just without the letters before my name (unless you count COB, GFE, PSE . . .).

Where would you learn about sex more: by complet-ing a university degree in sex, or by actually having it with a multitude of men from all backgrounds? Men are more honest when they're naked and vulnerable than they are in a drab meeting room with a candle and box of tissues in the corner. I would put money on the fact that I hear more honest confessions from husbands than any marriage coun-sellor would.

Samantha

Samantha was making fantastic money, having fantastic orgasms at work. How many of you orgasm at work? And guys, wanking in the toilet doesn't count.

I was earning more in three days as a sex worker than I was in one month as journalist for a national magazine. And more importantly, my job was giving me something more precious than money: time.

My days as a journalist involved too much rushing around, trying to fit my kids' school schedules into my own busy work week. I wasn't being a great mother and I wasn't being a great employee. I wasn't doing either job very well. My kids were frustrated and missed me, while my bosses and colleagues, though bloody patient, could see that I was being pulled between two different commitments. I felt guilty all the time. I was never in the office and I was always harassed with the kids.

But now they had their mummy back! We could have a coffee on the way to day care or kindy. I could pick them up early and we'd play in the park before getting ice-cream on the way home. I was present and I was focused. I had the time to attend the odd school trip, or to volunteer. And however hard the next sentence may be hard for you to comprehend, it's the truth. But being a sex worker made me a *better parent*.

It also had a dark side. Like any job, it's not perfect, and it would be disingenuous of me to glamourise it.

I started out as a day girl, but it was hard not to get drawn into the allure of the night-time shifts. The money was better, the doorbell went more frequently and it was a blast. The booze flowed, the music pumped and the chatter was a few notches higher too.

I started to work a few nights. I'd get home at 3 am, 4 am, once even past 5 am. The shifts were fun and lucrative, but the temptation to lose yourself in the moment was there, slyly inviting you in to join the party. The minibar looked so inviting at midnight when your drunk client was encouraging you to drink with him. And his cigarettes looked so inviting when you had a drink in your hand. And the drugs were available from clients if you wanted them, of course. Mostly to help you stay awake more than anything else. But they dulled your senses, took your control away, and that wasn't a safe place to be. You also risked being fired if management found out.

I remember having a threesome with a New Zealand girl, Hattie, and a Lebanese man. He was off his face on I don't know what, and we were helping him celebrate his birthday. The three of us jumped into the spa and somehow during our conversation the subject of Gorbachev, the ex-Soviet leader, came up. Hattie and I then decided it would be hilarious if we did a funny dance, naked, covered in suds, tapping our heads, singing out Gorbachev's name.

There was no sex, no debauched gang-bang. Just Hattie and I coping the best way we knew how in a three-hour booking with a pasty, overweight, wasted man – with humour. I went home that night concerned. I'd spent the day dancing naked chanting 'Gorbachev' with a naked Kiwi woman and a bemused Lebanese man. Was I losing the plot or just coping with a bizarre situation? Whatever the reason, I certainly didn't want to make a habit of it.

Another time I had to stay in a room for six hours with three young rich men and two other girls. The men were hot-shot bankers who snorted cocaine like it was going out of fashion. I paired up with one of them and had to spend at least half of that time trying to work a drugged up, flaccid penis. This was mentally draining work. It took my utmost willpower to not put my dress back on and walk out of the room. It was only back at home, when I was counting out the wads of green notes, that I could convince myself the six-hour session was only a small price to pay.

If I'd carried on with night shifts, my health would have suffered, for sure. I was always tired and a bit ratty the day after a big night shift. My head was full of ridiculous chatter from the night before. There were young handsome men from wealthy eastern suburbs families jumping on beds while naked and playing air guitar, and handing out credit cards that lasted all night. Or sneaky husbands who told their wives they were out for pizza and a beer with mates, only to ditch the pizza and come to The Bordello with excited eyes and hard cocks. Sometimes businessmen from overseas would make bookings at night after their day of meetings and stress. What better way to unwind than with a lovely lady, a beer and a spa to get naked in? They'd come in and choose two girls, or three or four of five. Maybe six! It was raucous, it was fun and it was all quite frankly a bit of a blur.

The night shifts were great but they took a toll. But even when I switched to just day shifts, I was usually too mentally drained to do anything socially, especially with friends I hadn't told about my job. I didn't like dishonesty, so spinning some bullshit about my whole working week to a friend would have been hard. I simply avoided people I'd chosen not to tell. I preferred they think I was unsociable rather than a liar.

My social life slowly disappeared, my interest in being in a relationship went and I began to feel disconnected from real life, most of all from myself.

Samantha loved having sex. She could have sex with anybody. Before Samantha came along, Amanda loved hanging out with guys, going on dates, the frisson of a first kiss. But now there was no point. The romantic chase no longer sparked my interest. It was like reading magazines for fun when I worked in magazines or having a facial when I was a beauty editor. It felt too much like work. The novelty had dissipated. A date with a man felt like another day in my 'office'.

I certainly didn't need men for sex, or for company. I was getting enough of both at work. So whenever a man asked me out, I would quite often say no. What would be the point? Was he using me for sex? Was I just another pussy to stick his penis in? Yawn.

And of course with that dangerous – and probably unfair – attitude, my sex life dried up, along with my social life. Most nights were me at home alone, taking off my make-up from the day's work, walking the dogs and going to bed early.

I questioned long-term, monogamous relationships. I often wondered how couples who had been married 40 years managed to do it. I certainly admired them. But the bullshit line, 'it's give and take', didn't wash with me anymore. It was more likely code for, 'He shagged a few birds along the way and I turned a blind eye.'

I worked part-time only for the best part of two years, and I saw a lot. I watched high-profile men smoking suspicious-looking pipes in the middle of the day before going home to their unsuspecting wives. I heard jaded young men despair at their lives and confide in me about how sick they were of cooking meals for one. There were so many great single women out there, and now all these single men. Why the hell weren't they finding each other? Were they looking in all the wrong places? Were they all so bitter? Or were they looking for the wrong things?

At my local café once, over scrambled eggs and sourdough, I happened to be seated next to a client. It was a situation neither of us relished. And to make matters even worse, he was sitting with his lovely, beaming family: a wife and three children. Absolutely bloody brilliant. Not only did I feel mortified that a client was in the same café as me, but also a client who'd last seen me in suspenders and a corset was now confronted by the sight of me in a Bonds tracksuit with greasy hair.

I turned and faced the other way, and he, no doubt, went paler than the whites of his eggs. It was a man I'd seen only one time, but I knew he was a regular at The Bordello and all the girls had been with him at least once.

I gazed at his family in the reflection of the window – his petite and beautiful wife and his well-behaved, adorable daughters in their dresses from Seed, with their hot chocolates and buttery banana bread. To the ordinary, untainted person, they might have looked such a lovely, happy family. Something we all strived for, and hoped existed.

Not to me. I could see the poison ivy creeping up between them. I knew his secrets. I knew he liked snorting coke off the perky breasts of 23-year-olds on Friday nights. I knew he would stay at The Bordello for six, seven hours at a time, that every hour he would change girls. Sometimes he brought work colleagues or friends along, even his brother-in-law once. There was a lot of that male camaraderie: the pack mentality.

The image was ruined for me. I didn't judge this man – who am I to judge someone else? I didn't know or care what else was going on in his life. But I judged marriage.

One of my young clients, whom I saw just the one time, had just come back from Las Vegas having experienced his first taste of wild abandonment. The only problem was he had got married not even six months ago. Las Vegas ignited a kind of freedom, some kind of need to root around on his poor wife. 'I'm just going to get it all out of my system and then I'll be faithful in six months' time,' he told me, before proceeding to peel my panties off with his teeth. I knew better.

Another young man paid me a visit the night before his wedding. Did he think in 24 hours' time he would no longer want to have sex with other women? I knew once that line was crossed, once the boundary was broken, you could forget it. Your marriage was never the same. What magic button did he think he was going to press? There was no STOP SHAGGING AROUND button in his brain.

It's to do with willpower and opportunity. And with the sex industry as rampant as it is, it takes men a hell of a lot of willpower to walk past a brothel when they ain't getting much at home.

Here's my confession: I have seen a friend's husband a few times. She isn't really a friend; I don't have her mobile number and I'd never meet her for a coffee. But I know her and her husband.

'Number 3's picked you, Sam,' Roxy called out one evening.

I glanced up from my magazine. Number 3 chose *me?*

'Did she say Sam?' I asked another girl. She nodded.

Fuck. Number 3 was Kate's husband – I think. Kate from Adelaide who I'd met a few times. Nah, I thought, there's no way he would be ballsy enough to pick me . . .

'Yes, it's me,' he smiled, grabbing my waist as we walked upstairs. 'And you, Amanda! How long have you worked here, you naughty thing? I saw your photos online, wow, you look great! I had to come in and see you. I hope you don't mind . . .'

I forced a smile. I was so good at faking these days. But I didn't like this. This wasn't kinky or sexy. It was over-stepping boundaries. It was uncomfortable enough that he was calling me Amanda. Don't call me Amanda here. This is Samantha's office. All the girls he could have picked. And he chose me. Fucking prick.

'Look, I don't really think we should do this –' I protested, but he pulled me close.

'Five hours,' he said pleadingly, passing me his credit card. 'I just want to talk.'

I raised my brow. What kind of confession was I going to get tonight? I knew Kate complained about her marriage sometimes, but what was I going to hear from her husband? And as you can imagine, there is a lot one can talk about in five hours in a room with a minibar.

'So – why?' I asked him, lighting his cigarette. 'What's wrong with your marriage? I mean, Kate, she seems so nice . . .'

'Of course she's nice,' he said. 'She's mother of our four kids but Amanda, I don't love her. I don't even like her. I've been coming here for over ten years. I've fucked over four hundred women and I've spent hundreds of thousands of dollars. When I think what that money could have gone towards – holidays for the kids, their education . . .' And he started to cry.

Jesus Christ, this was depressing. Poor bloody Kate, poor bloody him. I felt sorry for both of them, but I wasn't sure I really wanted to hear about it. I didn't want to intrude on their horrible, sad marriage. It was tiring enough knowing about the unhappy marriages of clients I wasn't friends with in real life. I didn't want to hear the ugly truth of people I knew.

'Hey, I'm really sorry,' I whispered, stroking his hair as he sniffed and wiped his eyes. 'But why don't you leave? Do her a favour and yourself one, and get a divorce?'

He looked at me, his eyes red and swollen. 'I just don't know that she will cope,' he whispered back. 'She needs me.'

I wasn't so sure. Would she rather have a husband who wasn't committed to the marriage just so there was someone to take the bins out? Or would she rather have been free to get on with her life and to meet someone who truly adored her? I knew which I would prefer. While her husband was in the wrong for wasting so much money in The Bordello, she probably had a part to play in all of this as well. Was her head so firmly deep in the sand that she couldn't see this happening, or didn't she care?

It was truly depressing. I left work with a heavy heart that night.

He kept coming back to see me, to talk it all through. I couldn't say no. I mean, who else was he going to talk to?

We never had sex and we barely even touched. I wasn't there for his wild and kinky sex fetishes. I was there as someone he could confess his sins to, and I didn't mind. I was glad he could talk to someone, even if it was someone who vaguely knew his wife. Maybe that's why he felt comfortable talking to me over a complete stranger.

He eventually stopped coming to see me. He was trying to 'be good' as he called it. I didn't see him again after that, and hoped that the two of them were able to work things out.

But how can I not take these experiences home with me? Were all marriages as sad as this? Were all men desperately lonely, were all women desperate to leave?

The more sad stories I heard at The Bordello, the lonelier I felt. Sometimes the old adage is true: that blissful ignorance is a better place to be.

A single woman always has that flicker of hope she will be whisked away by the love of her life. Wondering every day, 'Is this the day I'm going to meet Mr Right?'

That hope for me was burning out fast. Pah! Mr Right? Did he even exist? All the other women's Mr Rights were seriously unhappy in their marriages. What was the point in long-term relationships if no one was happy after a few years?

So yes, I saw a lot of lonely men at The Bordello. Men who would wait anxiously in the meeting rooms, not for a busty blonde to scoop them upstairs for dirty sex, but for a friendly woman who was a good listener to gently lead them to a quiet room to talk. And that always happened to be me.

One client in particular stays in my mind. His name was Locky, a big tough construction worker in his fifties. He looked like a tubby wrestler as he stomped up the stairs in his muddy Timberlands and neon-green worker's jacket. He ignored my trill of 'How's your day going?' and my pleasantries and simply grunted. A man of few words.

I was nervous. Locky was rough-looking. What kind of service could he want? I opened the door to one of the suites, letting him in before me. Could he be my first aggressive client?

Just as I closed the door behind me, I heard a sob. I spun round. It was coming from Locky. 'You're gunna need your tissues for this one, love,' he spluttered through his tears. 'I'm so sorry, this is embarrassing crying like this, but I didn't know where else to go.'

Before I had time to process the situation that was unfolding, Locky plonked his heaving body on the bed and put his head in his hands.

'I'm so sorry, love. I'm a bit of a mess.'

I handed him the box of tissues and sat beside him, stroking his back. 'It's all right, Locky, I've seen and heard it all before,' I replied softly. 'There's nothing to be ashamed of.'

'It's my wife,' he replied, cutting me off. 'I've just come back from the solicitor's. I signed off on the divorce.' And then he blew his nose into a clump of soggy tissues.

'I thought everything was going fine, until she told me out of the blue she was leaving. She'd met someone on Facebook. Michael. They were going to make a go of it, and she was moving to Tamworth to be with him. I've got three sons who live at home with me. The youngest is 15. I've never boiled an egg before, let alone put a load of washing on . . .'

I had to admit, even I was close to tears now. I hate seeing men cry, for starters, but to leave your kids? Your husband may be a pain in the arse, but to turn your back on your children? No, I could never do that.

'Oh Locky, I'm so sorry,' I replied, shaking my head and handing him more tissues. 'I'm sure you're a great father.'

'I don't want to make love, or anything, Samantha. I hope you're not too disappointed.' I smiled inwardly at his assumption.

'I have never been with any other woman besides Rita in 25 years. I probably wouldn't know what to do anyway. I've put on a few kilos now, and I wouldn't feel right taking my clothes off. I just needed to speak to someone,' he said, blowing his nose. 'It's hard being a man sometimes, love, we don't tend to talk as much as you sheilas do.' He looked at me, his eyes red and puffy, his nose covered in speckles of toilet tissue.

Poor Locky. How lonely he must have been feeling to come and pay $450 to break down in front of a stranger. He cried some more and then asked for my advice.

'Locky, if you want to know the truth, I think you need to get to the gym,' I said cautiously. 'Sign up today, right now, when you leave here. Get a personal trainer. Lose some weight, get fit, and meet new people. That's step number one.'

Locky looked up at me, nodding slowly.

'Then once you're feeling great, join a dating agency. Go on a few coffee dates, meet a few women, get your confidence back. It will take time, but it's something to look forward to. You need to move on from Rita. I don't think she will come back for you anytime soon.'

He left just as silently as he arrived but hopefully with a few so-called 'tools' under his belt. I hope I said the right thing to him, but I wasn't going to tell him to go to the pub, have a few beers and 'she'll be right, mate.'

Another client was a lovely Sri Lankan doctor with the softest, darkest skin I had ever touched. His parents had sent him to Sydney for a better life, where he studied medicine and became a success. He told me that he had no hope of meeting an Australian woman.

'I am ignored, Samantha, when I go to bars. Women walk past me with looks of arrogance or pity. If I start talking to an attractive lady, she scans the room for someone else to talk to, someone with white skin maybe. Or she will talk to me like I am stupid, because I am from Sri Lanka. It's only when I tell them I am a doctor that they hang around. If I mention that I drive a Mercedes, they decide they want to talk to me.

I don't want to come to The Bordello for sex. I want to meet someone in the real world. I want to have a wife and family. But I'm beginning to think that will never happen because of the colour of my skin.'

I felt a little bit ashamed. Was Australia still like this?

I had wiped the tears of so many men in those rooms. Their simplicity might have been too complex for us, but their vulnerability was not.

And income didn't seem to factor in when it came to these men's unhappiness. Greg inherited a fortune and didn't have to work. He was young, maybe only 30 and handsome. He lived in a mansion on the water, and drove one of his many sports cars into the Bordello car park probably four or five times a week.

He'd tell me about his day, which usually consisted of having lunch in a fancy restaurant somewhere, and not much else. He would lie on his back, close his eyes and say, 'I'm bored. Entertain me.'

'What do you do for work, Greg?' I asked him during our first session as I oiled his back.

'Nothing,' he replied, in a dull voice, not even opening his eyes.

'Nothing? What do you do all day?'

'Nothing. I'm bored.'

'Why don't you start up a charity, or go overseas?'

'Yeah, nah. Boring.'

'Meet a girl, have a baby?'

'Boring.'

'Go out with mates?'

'They're always working. Boring.'

Our session was always boring. Afterwards, Greg would

132

have a shower, put his clothes on slowly, and say something about the weather outside being 'shit' so he would just go home and do nothing.

Greg's wealthy lifestyle may seem enviable to some, but let me tell you, having too much money can be very isolating – and can make people extremely dull. Greg clearly had no purpose. I would guess that he suffered depression and lacked drive.

It doesn't matter whether you're CEO of a bank or a mechanic. You all speak the same words and feel the same emotions.

Strength comes from admitting your weaknesses and fragility.

You men may not tell each other how tough you're doing it, or how lonely and depressed you're be feeling, but I wish you would, because there is one person you are confiding in – and that's me.

AMANDA
Discovering Lola's

Search 'Boutique Brothels Sydney' or 'High Class Girls Sydney' in Google and you'll get pages and pages of escort agencies, parlours and erotic massage places. How did I come to end up where I did? It's not like there's any recruitment agency and there is certainly no one to advise you. Who would you ask, anyway?

After my experiences as a single woman in Sydney, and particularly after my rendezvous with Matthew the married man, I had decided that this was it. The time was now. My toe-dipping into the dark world had to stop. It was time to dive in.

I was still working three days a week in the office and loved my job, but something wasn't right for me anymore. I'd lost my passion – for that career anyway. I was bored. I needed something fresh. Something exciting. I wanted to stop writing other people's stories and instead create my own.

That lovely house with the frangipani tree . . . I just couldn't get it out of my mind. I knew exactly where it was, which street, which number. It had been years since the incident with the abusive woman, and now, after my marriage had ended, I would drive past occasionally and look up, wondering.

The need to investigate, as a journalist, was always there. I had to get to bottom of everything. I lived my life on a need-to-know basis and as it just so happened, I needed to know everything. So when it came to the sex industry and the secretive world of men and sex, I was fascinated. Call it research, an investigation or curiosity. But I had to find out about that beautiful home with the white shutters and the tree.

I just had to call them and make an appointment; easy as that.

Except it wasn't. I punched in 'discreet brothel xxxx street' but nothing came up. I tried mixing the words round, still nothing. Again and again I tried, but that lovely little place with the mad woman living next door had seemingly disappeared.

One spring day, I drove to that house, parked outside and knocked on the door, my curiosity getting the better of me. I noticed the same Lexus parked next door and braced myself for another barrage of abuse. The mad woman was clearly still there.

No answer, so I knocked again. A pregnant woman in her thirties with glowing skin and designer clothes opened the door. 'Hello?' she smiled warmly.

'Oh!' I replied, not expecting this. 'Sorry, do you live here?'

My eyes quickly scanned the hallway for signs of secret sex. But there was an umbrella stand, polished floorboards, photos of a happy family, and kids' Crocs neatly tucked under a table. If this was a brothel, and this pregnant lady a madam, I would be very, very surprised.

'Yes I do,' she said, waiting for my explanation. 'Sorry, I've got the stove on . . . can I help you?'

'Sorry,' I mumbled, turning away, slightly embarrassed. 'I must have got the wrong house.'

'That's fine,' replied the woman, again smiling at me – almost knowingly. *Looking for the brothel, were we?* I could almost hear her thoughts.

Well I could cross that one off my list. It clearly had either moved or didn't exist. Maybe that red-haired woman, whose Lexus was almost grinning at me now, was simply stark raving mad. Or maybe I was – did I imagine the whole thing?

Instead of forgetting my ridiculous idea of research, this only made me more determined. I called every phone number that looked slightly close, but nothing sounded right, nothing sounded me. Eventually, just as I was about to throw it all in, I dialled the number of a place named Lola's. It was right in the hustle and bustle of the northside business district. They had no proper website, just the name 'Lola's' and a number. That alone sparked my interest.

The woman on the end of the phone was soft-spoken and polite.

'Why don't you come in for a chat?' she said. 'I'll give you the address on the day, if you don't mind.'

This was still research, as far as I could tell. I told myself this as I drove through the city. Purely research.

Lola's was discreet, an upmarket and boutique penthouse atop a high-rise in North Sydney. The madam was Nina.

'You'll do very well here,' Nina said, as I sat in front of her nervously. She was in her late fifties, tanned and attractive, with short dark hair and a tiny figure. She wore a leopard print and black outfit and smart black shoes with a slight kitten heel. Her nails were a luscious dark cherry.

'Tea?' she offered, clicking across the kitchen tiles. 'I'm afraid I don't have any biscuits to offer you. The girls polished off the Tim Tams on the weekend; those nice caramel-centred ones. What with that rain, it was so quiet here, there wasn't much else to do.'

We immediately bonded. She told me how she grew up in Africa, but had settled in Sydney. Her love for Africa was still visible; she liked her leopard print and African artefacts, like the tall wooden giraffe I'd spotted in the corner. 'I miss the horizon, the people,' she said during our conversation, her voice trailing off sadly.

I liked her enormously. 'I've been here 12 years,' she said. 'Business has tailed off a bit now. We've had to move three times and yes I'll admit it, we lost a few of the clientele from doing that. Men don't like too much change, you see. And it doesn't help that the parking is atrocious around here. I hope you found somewhere? Oh I do hope you don't get a ticket. Awful people, those parking police. Why they don't get proper jobs I'll never know.'

The phone rang, which she answered immediately. 'No, I told you already, Jack, Hannah is no longer working here. No I don't know where she's gone. That's fine, Jack, do what you must . . .'

Nina looked and me and rolled her eyes. 'Doddery old geriatric fellow,' she whispered to me, covering the mouthpiece with her hand, '75 years old, likes to sail. We call him Popeye.'

I smiled. He sounded like quite a character. Looking around the modest but homey décor, it was almost as though I could have been sitting in the living room with my mum, our feet up, drinking Earl Grey. Except that the relationship with my mother was at the best of times silent, and at worst nasty.

Often I thanked God I had Tab's mum, Veronica, whom I called my surrogate mother. During my heart ordeal, and even through my divorce, she would come with me to hospital appointments or call me to check up on me in general. 'You're doing a great job, sweetheart,' she would reassure me if I had a bad day with the kids.

And with Nina, I felt that connection too.

'It's $350 an hour, of which you'll get $200,' she said briskly, putting on her glasses – even they were leopard print. 'The clients here are lovely men; mostly older gentlemen, but very nice. I mean, they can be annoying sometimes, and they're not always the most attractive of fellows, but they're harmless. We have two other girls working here, Mary and Trish. You'll meet them soon. Do you have any questions?'

'What about weirdos or serial killers? Or the police?' I asked. Well I had to ask – I was a journalist after all – I had to ask.

Nina peered at me from under her specs. 'My dear,' she said, smiling, 'you've been watching too much TV. Nothing exciting has ever happened here!'

Then she took a sip of tea. 'Why did you choose Lola's?' she asked. 'We hardly advertise these days. I keep telling the boss to create some sort of internet thingy, a website, but I think he's lost interest in the place.'

'Look, I'll be honest,' I replied. 'I was actually looking for a place down the road. It looked like a lovely home and there was a frangipani tree outside and a mad redheaded woman living next door . . .'

Nina put her cup down and looked at me. I'd got her attention.

'. . . I was standing on a street corner opposite this house, years ago, and this woman just started screaming at me that I was a hooker. Obviously I wasn't, and I just thought I must have been standing outside a brothel. Anyway, it looked so lovely, that house, I mean so warm and friendly, that I thought if I was going to work as an escort, I would like to start there. I've been trying to find it, but I think I must have got it wrong. That woman was obviously mad, or I was, I'm not quite sure yet.'

'Gosh, she's still there,' Nina murmured quietly, shaking her head in disbelief. 'We called her The Dragon. She was a frightful woman. That was us, dear. That beautiful home was Lola's. That woman, you're right, is mad, utterly mad. She hated the fact she bought a house next door to a brothel. But we never made a sound. We were always so respectful of our neighbours, but she terrorised us. Kept sending her poor husband in to catch us out. That poor fellow. Anyway, we moved a few years ago now; some young family moved in . . .'

I didn't hear the rest of her words. I was merely watching her mouth move. My search had taken me to the very place I'd been looking for all along.

Do you ever get a feeling some things are just meant to be?

Chapter Ten

AMANDA

A storm

So that was it. I was sold. A big believer in my angels opening the doors for me, I knew that finding Lola's was a sign that it was all meant to be. My angels didn't just guide me, they led me right to the front bloody door. So here I was. Amanda was going to become a call girl! It was so ... well ... petrifying. But after my experience with Mr Burns and Nice Dentist and even Bad Breath (Nina was always spot on with her descriptions), I settled into my new role easier than expected. You know when you curl your toes around the fluffy insides of your ugg boots (or in my case nine-inch heels)? It felt like I was home.

When I first began working as a call girl, I worked for Nina only two days a fortnight. On the other days I worked as a journalist or spent the day with my kids. But I increasingly started to look forward to my Samantha days.

Nina was right: Lola's was quiet. Business was slow. Most of the clients were over 55 – one was past 80 – but they were all old-fashioned gentlemen. It was a miracle no one had a heart attack on my watch. But it was a great place to learn the ropes, to ease myself in to the performance I was now required to master. It was in fact the perfect place to learn a lot of things.

I learnt to read men quickly using the little clues they leave around, from their clothes (unflattering baggy jeans were a good indicator he was a dad), to what they wanted (someone to cuddle, mostly). I realised that men didn't like to be rough in bed; really, they wanted slow, intimate sex. They want foreplay – lots of it – and they loved giving oral. That's right, *giving*. Sometimes, as I lay back in bliss, I could hardly believe that I was being paid to have orgasms.

The single men were simply grateful to be holding a naked woman and wanted the whole thing to last as long as possible.

I learnt that men want to pleasure you, to adore you, to make sure you're satisfied and happy. Many of my clients came in asking, 'How can I make you happy?' (It was tempting not to reply: 'By leaving your money on the bed and walking out the front door again.')

And I was shocked to learn that notion that men can't multi-task is absolute rubbish. My theory is that we were brainwashed into believing this by lazy men who just didn't want to take out the bins while they were watching the cricket. These men were in fact very good multi-taskers. Every single one of them could kiss, touch, stroke, fuck, and talk all at once. Some could even swig a beer or smoke at the same time. There was one arrogant young man who visited me once – no older than 20 – who smoked a cigarette the whole time I was bouncing up and down on his cock with faux pleasure.

He even answered his mobile and spoke to his girlfriend while staring at me the whole time. The urge to rip out his cigarette and stub it on his tip of his nose was too overwhelming. 'I have to pee,' I muttered, climbing off. What a jerk.

I learnt that being a worker made me feel more in control of my situation. Having grown men in awe of my body was something I wasn't used to these days. It was flattering to see these clients returning week after week to see me. I must have been doing something right! I grew more confident with each shift; it was pretty hard not to when all you heard all day was, 'Wow, you're amazing' and, 'You're beautiful.' While I knew that some might argue it was all fantasy, I didn't care. I always felt happy when I left work. I felt good about myself, and I know that I made men feel good about themselves too. I had achieved something worthwhile. And so what if we were naked?

Nina and I would often sit and chat for hours between appointments. We became good friends. We'd laugh about the clients, and occasionally, when it was quiet (which it often was) she would find something nice in the fridge, like a Cloudy Bay, and crack it open for us to share.

'You're going to do extremely well, my dear,' she said once, handing me a glass one afternoon.

'Really?' I replied, slipping off my heels and plonking myself down on the well-worn black leather sofa. I'd been at Lola's just a few months – could she tell already?

'Oh yes – and don't let anyone tell you you're too old. You've got at least ten years of working in you, and damn, you make sure you make the most of it. Don't give it all up for a man.'

She took a large sip of wine and slammed the glass down, staring at me intently.

Nina was quite forceful about the idea of female independence. Not that she was anti-men, but I think she had trusted a few men in her life and had been let down.

You can see her charm, can't you? If you ever met her, you would fall in love with her too. She was maternal without being smothering and fun without being cringe-worthy. She was all class and to me, she was exactly how I thought a madam should be.

But back to age. Anyone who thinks women become invisible after the age of 50 hasn't been to Cougars, a brothel that specialises in older women. When I say specialises, I mean they offer mature women – exclusively.

When I went in there for an interview it was more to have a good nose at the place than to work there. It was fascinating. I sat by the cluttered reception waiting for the owner to find a spare minute to chat, and happily watched the real-life reality show that was unfolding in front of me.

I could not believe it. Women ranging from the ages of 40 to 70, dressed in lingerie and heels, were lined up in front of me waiting to meet clients in the introduction rooms.

There were women with all manners of bodies, blonde hair, greying hair, white hair. I saw one much older woman who had a slight hunch and folds of pale pasty flesh pouring out of her bra strap, yet she seemed to be one of the busiest ladies there.

Don't laugh or wrinkle your nose up – that doorbell went twice every minute. Men of all ages fast-paced it to the introduction room, their eyes lighting up with the feast of women in front of them. Normal men! (Well, they looked normal anyway.) The clients were a mix of older gents, tradies and especially younger men.

'Oh yes, most of our clientele are under 35,' Joan, the receptionist, told me, buzzing yet another man in through the front door. 'Our ladies are all very warm and friendly in the bedroom. No haughty princesses here.'

Cougars was far busier than Lola's and The Bordello.

Lola's on the other hand was dying. It had been booming back in the 90s, in the frangipani house, but the owners had other businesses to run and didn't want to spend any money on the place.

My regulars either couldn't afford to come every week or they got too old and died. The younger men seemed to be going elsewhere for sex.

Because I wasn't relying solely on Lola's for income, I was happy to treat the job as a bit of fun, an experiment, scratching an itch. And the extra cash was very, very welcome.

Then one blustery day that I was on-shift at Lola's, as branches of the palm trees blew almost to the ground and office workers were clasping their swaying umbrellas tightly, the unexpected happened. Busted by cops? A geriatric popped his clogs while doing doggie? Some old codger got stuck in the shower with his Zimmerframe? Nope.

The roof blew off.

Yep. It was a bad storm; the building was probably as old and rickety as some of the clients. A few tiles ripped off, then a few more, and they tumbled down to the pavement, barely missing the shocked, drenched commuters, leaving a gaping hole in the roof, and a mortified client covering his privates with the bed sheets. Lola's was exposed. The owners didn't want to pour cash into renovating. So it closed up shop for good.

Amanda

A few days afterwards I met Nina for a coffee. 'Well, I'm not quite sure what I'm going to do with myself,' she said, nursing a flat white. 'There's a part-time job going in a beauty salon, but darling – and you'll understand this – the owner is German, and we all know how cold they are. You must go on, though. You've got a great future ahead of you in this game, and by God darling, you jolly well take it by the horns!'

As dramatic as ever, she slammed her cup down and gave me one of her intent stares, as little drops of milky coffee splattered all over the red tablecloth.

But I wasn't so sure. Was this the end of my brief part-time career as Samantha? Was the ferocious storm an angry sign from my angels saying 'enough!'?

It should have been, but Samantha was just finding her feet. She hadn't just been born; she was alive and kicking. My angels would have to try a little harder than that.

SAMANTHA
Josh

One of the first things people always do when I tell them about my career is wrinkle their noses and say: 'Eurgh. What about the fat ugly men? Can't you say no to them?'

Well yes, I can say no to anyone I like. It is my body. But the thing is, unless they're rude or arrogant, I don't. I have only ever kicked out one client – a well-dressed businessman – and that was because he was rude to me. 'Have I done something to offend you, sir?' I asked him as I poured him a drink. 'Are you shy or just plain rude? Because I'm terribly sorry, but I do not see rude men.' His face dropped as I marched out of the room and slammed the door behind me. 'Roxy, can you deal with the twat in room 2? He ordered me around and I don't like him.'

'Of course, Samantha,' she replied briskly. 'I'll get rid of him.'

The nice clients are mostly unattractive ones and the good-looking clients are a massive pain in the arse. They're arrogant and expect you to throw in the kissing for free because they're so hot and cute, and aren't I lucky that they picked me . . .

But let me tell you about Josh, whom I saw only once, yet whose positivity and outlook on life stayed with me.

Josh had a handsome face. He had kind, brown eyes and messy, dark hair. He was smart, but his greatest asset was his sense of humour. From the minute we set eyes on each other, we were chatting like old friends.

He was probably in his thirties, sharp as a tack and witty as they come. I left our session with a happy glow inside, like I'd just been on a great date and the feeling was mutual. Josh would have made someone the perfect partner. Except for one thing.

Josh had brittle bone disease. His bones didn't form correctly in the womb, which meant that even a tiny knock could leave him reeling in pain. A little pressure in the wrong place could cause his fragile bones to snap like little twigs.

He was confined to a wheelchair and came to The Bordello with his personal carer, who had to lift him on the bed, help him into the shower, onto the toilet, then back on the bed. Pretty humiliating, some might think. But humiliation was something he was probably used to.

His arms and legs were like twisted chicken wings. Bone and skin painfully jutted out of his hugely deformed body.

Honestly, Josh was the most physically impaired human being I had ever seen. No matter how non-judgemental and open-minded you were, I promise you would take a sharp intake of breath at his appearance.

And he happened to wheel into The Bordello just as I was about to leave for the day.

'Samantha,' hissed Roxy quietly as I turned the key into my locker. 'There are a couple of men in the intro room. One's in a wheelchair, the other is his carer. They've been waiting for almost an hour. I know you're about to leave, and of course you can say no, but do you see disabled clients?'

Why was it always me doing the bloody favours? Sighing, I checked the time. It was ten to seven, and I was supposed to be leaving at 7 pm. 'Um . . .' I hesitated. I had no one to go home to, but did I see disabled clients? I hadn't ever, no . . . but could I?

'Thing is, the only other girl who would meet him isn't here. No one does disabled. Could you just meet him? Please?' she pleaded, looking slightly panicked about how to handle the situation.

I glanced at her. The poor guy had come to The Bordello and only one out of the nine girls there would meet him? He'd been sitting there, humiliated, for almost an hour, knowing that he couldn't even pull a root in a brothel?

'Of course I'll meet him,' I replied, taking my key out. 'That's fine, Roxy. Just let me freshen up first.'

I could tell she wanted to hug me (hey, that's $50 Roxy!). 'You're a star,' she grinned. 'Thank you.'

But how could I not agree to meet this man? How embarrassed, how humiliated he must feel waiting there patiently, stuck on his steel prison, for a girl to be introduced to. And to hear all the girls chatting and carrying on in the changing room, knowing that he repelled them.

I could never judge the other girls I worked with, but I do judge myself. It didn't sit right with me to leave him there. It didn't feel okay to me to turn someone down because he was in a wheelchair. He was brave enough to come to this intimidating brothel with his carer, and face the stares and shocks of pretty girls, and someone had to be brave enough to spend time with him.

The way I saw it, I was a sex worker. My job was to give men an intimate special time, and in return for that, they paid me. I couldn't discriminate against someone for the colour of their skin, or the body they were in. I felt strongly that every single one of us is entitled to a sex life. If you couldn't have sex in a brothel, then where the hell were you supposed to go?

When I drew back the curtain and met Josh for the first time, I was hoping against hope that the shock wasn't written all over my face. And if it was, Josh, I apologise.

He was basically a torso in a wheelchair. His hands looked like they were attached to his shoulders and his feet looked like they were attached to his hips. He didn't have arms and he had small twisted legs. He was a bit like a ball – except he wasn't fat. He actually had a nice chest and a friendly face.

His carer, George, looked like he belonged in a bikie gang, wearing a tight black T-shirt stretched over a podgy tummy, black jeans and a nose-ring. But he had a kind face and was protective over his patient. He eyed me up cautiously and I knew what he was thinking: 'Please don't fuck this up.'

'Let me guess which one needs the shag more,' I quipped bravely. 'George. You look like you haven't been laid in years!'

Josh laughed out loud and George nearly spat out his chewing gum. Ice broken.

'I'd get up and shake your hand, except you may have noticed I don't have legs and my hands are a bit crap,' joked Josh. 'So why don't you come and sit beside me and we can have a quick chat before I decide over the plethora of women who wanted to meet me today.'

'Josh, I'm sorry –'

'Hey – no need to apologise, Samantha. Their loss! I'm sure you'll tell them all what a great root I was.'

'So Josh, are you in full working order?'

'Yes.'

'And what kind of service are you looking for today?'

'Look,' he said, nodding at George to light him a cigarette. 'I just want to be with a woman who makes me laugh and who doesn't treat me like a leper. I get that enough in the real world. I want a few drinks, a few fags and a shag, but most importantly, good conversation and a laugh. Reckon you're up for the challenge?' And he looked at me with a twinkle in his eye.

'Bloody oath I am, Josh, question is, is biker boy over there going to sit and watch, because you can pay double if he is!'

Of course biker boy wasn't going to watch. He was there to assist in the admin of it all. I left the room while he helped Josh shower and eased him onto the bed. He was then given instructions to return in one hour.

I'll be honest. I was shitting myself. I was absolutely terrified. How the fuck was Samantha going to go with this one? Was I supposed to twirl around like a porn star with a man who couldn't touch me? I closed my eyes and muttered a prayer to my angels, who were probably loving every moment of this circus.

As I swung open the door, I put on the happiest, most excited face I could muster. 'Are you ready, handsome?' I sang, stepping in.

'Well don't just stand there staring at my gorgeous hunk of a body, pour us some drinks and light me a cigarette, will ya?' smiled Josh. 'And then we'll talk about taking your clothes off.'

The hour went fast. Josh was a funny, smart, totally together man.

We lay on the bed together, drinking and sharing stories, and covered subjects from his disease to his work. I don't recall the words so much but I remember we laughed a lot.

But jokes aside, I wanted to get an idea of his life. What was it like living in that . . . *shell?*

'I was born like this,' he said, taking a drag of his cigarette. 'I'm used to this – it's other people who need to get used to me. I see their eyes when I go past them in the street, disgust and horror at the way I look. They can't help themselves; I get it. I heard a little boy ask his mum what was wrong with "that man". His mum was really awkward about it, tried to shut him up. I wheeled over, and told her it was okay. I explained to the kid that something was wrong with my body and I didn't have the same limbs as him, but I had the same brain. If we teach kids not to be scared of us, hopefully then they'll make less judgemental, less fearful adults.'

He talked about wanting to meet someone one day, to settle down. 'But only when I'm ready, and only with the right person. They have to make me laugh,' he said. The person he ended up with would be a lucky woman.

The sex was, in all honesty, awkward. 'Just tell me if I hurt you,' I warned him, climbing gently on top of his little body. It could hardly be passionate and steamy; it was more of a carefully executed operation.

Just as we getting into the swing of things, and I was gently squatting over him, he let out a scream. 'Ow, my leg,' he winced, rubbing his tiny leg.

'Oh my God, what?' I yelped, climbing off.

'It's okay, my leg is just in pain.'

'Shit, have I broken your leg?'

'You may have, I'm not sure,' he croaked, rubbing it fiercely.

'Should I call George? Should I call reception?' My panic was rising. Had I just made things worse for him?

The pain thankfully subsided and we tried again. This time I sat Josh up against the pillows and went on all fours behind him. As we made love, I could see the reflection of his face in the mirror, his sheer bliss. If there ever was to be a man in heaven, it was Josh right there. And without wanting to sound like Mother friggin' Teresa, it made me feel good.

If I was to go on a date, give me Josh any day. He had more drive, more passion and more courage than any man I'd met. He was cursed with a terrible disease but was also blessed with a spirit and a heart that made him unique.

He managed a sly sort of self-deprecation without the self-pity. He made me see that you really can't judge someone by their body and their looks, and that really, the nicest souls are inside the bodies we least expect them to be.

'The disabled goddess now, eh, Roxy?' I grinned, nudging Roxy on my way to the girls' room.

'You betcha, Sam,' she said, winking.

It was my experience with Josh that saw my online profile on The Bordello website expand, another feather to my bow on my sex CV. Not only did I now 'specialise in couples', but also 'disabled' clients.

Chapter Eleven

AMANDA
Love in the real world

A gorgeous man tried to pick me up while I was walking my dogs. I'd seen him around my local area. Mmm, I'd think as he walked past, smiling at me, holding my gaze. He was exactly my type: stocky, dark hair, dark eyes and big, big arms.

We had never got further than a few eye flutters (me not him) until today. 'Hey,' he said casually as he sauntered up to me. I was sitting on some grass, watching the ocean with my dogs. 'I'm Jake.' He extended his muscly tanned arm, and as I shook his giant hand, I felt myself getting a bit giddy inside. Was he coming over to chat me up? *Me?*

He sat down on the grass next me and didn't seem to have any intention of leaving anytime soon. He was 35, worked as a designer, and lived locally. 'But I have Fridays off,' he said, his dark eyes twinkling. 'How about we meet next Friday? I'm always bored on Fridays.' He lived close by, he said.

I gave him my email address and walked off, excited. I liked Jake. He was handsome, confident and open. Could he be my next boyfriend? He ticked all the boxes and I liked meeting men in day-to-day situations. Since I'd begun working as Samantha, men seemed to approach me more. Did I give off some kind of sexual scent? I didn't dress any differently, but had started carrying myself better. Shoulders back, tits out kind of thing. After all, men were parting from their hard-earned cash to spend time with me. I couldn't be that bad could I?

And right on cue, Jake emailed barely an hour later. Gosh, he was keen. I liked it! A man who didn't play games . . .

And here is what he wrote:

Hi Amanda,
Was nice meeting you today at the beach . . . Would be nice to catch up for a coffee and have a chat, tomorrow if you are free?
As it is better to be up front, I'd like to let you know I am married. However, I hope it is still ok for a coffee.
Ciao,
Jake.

Hang on. Say again?

As it is better to be up front, I'd like to let you know I am married.

Married. ***Married.*** **MARRIED!!**
Excuse my obvious DUMBNESS, my blaring naivety, but didn't we just spend the good part of an hour TALKING face

to face, eye to eye? Didn't Jake have plenty of time and opportunity to tell me he was married? Maybe when he stroked my arm or when he pointed out my goosebumps, or took his sunnies off to meet my eyes; or when he went on about HIS unit's renovations, and how HE chose this and HE chose that; how much he loves meeting new people, how he loves English girls and how BORED he gets on Fridays ... silly him, he forgot to tell me he had a wife at home.

The cheeky fuck wanted exactly that every Friday. So this is what I typed back:

> *Dear Jake,*
> *That's ok. Thank you for being honest. I'm pretty honest too.*
> *I am a high-class escort. If you would like to have a sexual*
> *relationship, we can come to some arrangement.*
> *Thanks,*
> *Amanda.*

He made some pathetic reply about how he 'wasn't expecting that' and could we 'still meet for coffee' but I couldn't be arsed. He was living in a cramped one-bedroom unit with his long-suffering wife. He probably couldn't even afford me.

I read many memoirs by other call girls and they seemed to go on about how much they hated men, about how they'd now become lesbians and seen the light.

Actually, I don't agree. Men are selfish, sure. They don't just want their cake, they want an all-you-can-eat buffet. But I don't hate them. It's a bit like hating crying babies on a long-haul flight, or a puppy that has just chewed your Louboutins. Hate isn't the right word. It's too cruel.

It's closer to pity and frustration at these blundering fools. It can't be nice wandering around town all day being governed by a penis. Seriously, with a small flaccid piece of flesh with one dribbling eye as your master, it can't be very empowering.

My theory is that most men don't act with malice. That puppy didn't chew your shoes out of spite. He just couldn't help himself.

I began to understand men a bit better than I used to, which is why I changed my approach to real-life dating. I suppose I felt more confident in myself. I knew men reacted well to blunt honesty. And I didn't take crap from men in my real world anymore. Would the old Amanda have met Jake for a coffee? Probably! And she would have done it out of boredom and to get laid. But in my double life as Samantha, those needs were being met. My life was far from boring and my sex life was certainly active. I didn't need men when I had Samantha.

One-night stands were another thing that fell by the wayside when Samantha was born. I just could not be bothered. More so, I felt I was worth more. Not in monetary value, but I refused to let myself be used by men anymore.

Clients sometimes asked me if I had a boyfriend. I'd always say no, even if I happened to have one at the time. Partly, I didn't want to picture his lovely face during my appointments, but mostly, clients would rather think I was single. It would have interfered with the fantasy they were paying me for if I were to hint at my romantic life outside work. I dated a few men and I told them what I did for a living, much to the horror of my other working girlfriends. Even the girls I worked with who lived with their boyfriends told them they worked as a nanny or in an office – God knows how they got away with that. I marvelled at their ability to carry on the charade without being eaten up with guilt. But what did I know? It'd been years since I'd lived with a partner. Maybe the rules were different for those younger girls – or maybe the young men they were living with just couldn't have handled the truth.

But lying didn't agree with me. It fucked with my head. When you lie to everyone about everything, you can't keep track of which lie you've told each person. It's better to simply tell the truth, right?

Yeah, great advice. Except that my boyfriend was a cop. The lovely and muscly Dan, from somewhere out west, was a law-abiding, law-enforcing police officer. He rightly assumed I worked on a magazine (I was doing my three days a week there at the time) but I didn't tell him about the other two days at The Bordello.

So I kept my mouth shut, guiltily. Every time he did something nice it felt like torture. If he knew the truth, he wouldn't love the real me, that's for sure. Or at least that's what I believed. When he offered to take me to work on one occasion, I froze. It was a Thursday, my day at The Bordello. 'No, honey, it's fine,' I replied briskly, changing the subject to how lovely the jacarandas were this time of year.

'I'll pick you up at 8,' he said, kissing my forehead. 'I'll bring you a coffee.' Shit. I couldn't argue with a police officer, could I?

So what did I do? The poor bastard drove me 30 minutes out of his way to my magazine office, his hand entwined with mine the whole time, while I sat there with my stomach in twisting, cramping, guilt-laden knots, with sweat pouring out of my head, feeling light-headed and sick. Every time he stopped at a red light it took every bit of strength in me not to either open the door and throw myself out or turn round and say, 'I'm sorry, I'm a hooker.' I hated this deceit. It wasn't fair to Dan. How did people live double lives? I couldn't even have a double journey to work. I'd never been so happy to see the depressingly sterile magazine offices as we pulled up outside. I leapt out of the car and walked through the glass doors and into the reception, much to the bemusement of my colleagues, who didn't expect me in till Monday. 'Just picking something up,' I mouthed to them, pretending to press the button for the elevator.

I waved Dan off and hovered around the reception area with nervy stomach cramps, biting my French-manicured nails, waiting till he became a very faint dot in the distance. Then I jumped in a taxi to The Bordello, feeling very guilty and with a bad tummy for the rest of the day. And that is why lying will always be a complete headfuck for me.

Anyway, you'd think that being a cop he might have cottoned on. He might have noticed the array of crotchless panties and all-in-one neon-pink teddies hanging on my washing line. Or my nine-inch 'stripper' heels that I only put on for him *in* bed. There was also the fact that I knew how to put on a condom with my mouth which might have aroused suspicion, and that I happily gave him massages post-ejaculation as if it were the most natural thing in the world. Nope. When I confessed, Dan was shocked.

'I just don't understand why you have to do this,' he said tearfully, shaking his head. 'Why do such a soul-destroying job? It's so dangerous, Amanda. I care about you, you don't need to do this . . .'

I felt a surge of anger inside. Didn't he understand? Of course I didn't *have* to do this. Of course I didn't *need* to. I was not on the breadline. I was not some kind of victim, or abused, or an alcoholic or drug addict. Sure, I had a crap relationship with my mother, but who doesn't have some kind of story? I was a sex worker because (and here's something you may have guessed by now) I enjoyed it.

Some of you will not believe me. You'll think that deep down I have a self-loathing issue, that I feel I'm worth nothing more to anyone than a quick fuck. Or you think I have serious mental issues and I am scarred or unhinged. Maybe you agree with an ex-boyfriend of mine, who told me, 'All prostitutes have psychological problems.'

Don't we all, though? Who at some stage of their life hasn't had a 'psychological issue'? You certainly don't need to be wearing a beaded pearl thong to have had one.

There must be something wrong with me! I'd have to be terribly insecure or a raving lunatic to want to be paid for sex.

Er, not exactly. I hate to break it to you, but I am actually pretty normal. I have a counsellor, which I deem a luxury. Doris is a wonderful lady and keeps me in check. Sometimes I walk in feeling like a mess, and walk out feeling centred. Sometimes I cry about my mother, other times we laugh about my clients. I always secretly admire her pedicures and nice clothes, and I often wonder what she makes of me. But that hour, that golden hour once a week, is precious. It's my time. I don't have to listen to anyone's issues apart from mine.

I'm not perfect, I struggle with a few things. But come on, who doesn't?

Doris knows I'm torn between feeling like I shouldn't be doing my job because it's 'wrong' and feeling guilty because I actually enjoy it. Through our sessions, I learnt to finally admit that I preferred having a man pay hundreds of dollars to have sex with me for one hour instead of sitting in front of a computer in a boxy office all day, and that this was okay.

But Dan didn't understand that, and I was too kind to spell it out to him.

Seeing him cry stirred something in me beneath my anger: guilt. So I stopped working. 'I'm going on a holiday,' I told Roxy reluctantly, who was of course understanding. I'm sure she'd heard it a million times before.

'Sure, Sammy. You just let me know when you're back and ready to rock and roll.'

At first, it was actually quite nice having a boyfriend. I cooked him organic eggs and bacon in the morning when he was up early for his shift. We would sit on a park bench (me on his lap) and watch the boats gently sway in the harbour until the sun went down. But our moments of time together were few and far between – small snatches of sex and love in-between his shifts and my being with the kids. I was spending a lot of time alone, missing him.

You know who else I missed? My dear friend, Samantha. I missed the cash, the sex and the fun. I wasn't seeing Dan much and I wasn't seeing Samantha. And I started to realise that going cold turkey on my job for a man I rarely saw was beginning to piss me off. I started to take it out on Dan. My bills weren't paying themselves.

'For God's sake, go back to work,' he snapped back one day. 'You've been depressed ever since you stopped.'

He lectured me on the amount of incidents he had to go to at parlours and brothels. 'I'm worried about your safety, but you're a grown woman,' he went on. I hopped skipped and jumped back into my heels but a few months later, Dan did the right thing and ended the relationship, saying I was 'on the path to destruction' and he had 'failed to save me'.

He was possibly correct. But I didn't feel I needed saving. I wasn't 24 years old; I was worldly. I was choosing this role as a professional, educated and smart woman. I was working the industry, it wasn't working me. *Saving?*

I was upset. No one likes being dumped. But I was also indignant. No, I did not need saving.

My next boyfriend after Dan was a paramedic. Can you see a pattern here? It wasn't the uniform I was attracted to, it was the feeling of being protected. I hadn't really had much of that in my life. My parents, as much as they did love me, always taught me fierce independence. 'You'll thank me one day when you don't rely on anyone,' Mum would say. At the time I thought it was her excuse for not wanting me around. It was, in her eyes, to teach me to stand up on my own two feet. But when it came to boyfriends, I looked for someone strong and protective. Whether he was a cop or a standover man, I didn't care. I just wanted to know that he could look after me physically. I always liked big arms for the way they feel wrapped around me, cocooning me from the world.

My paramedic was older, separated and I was honest with him from day one. 'I work at The Bordello,' I announced to him over a smoothie. His eyes lit up excitedly. He was great. Not only would he rush over to feed fluids into my arm when I was hungover, but he was fully supportive of my job.

'Amanda, if women wanted to pay me $450 for sex, I'd bloody jump at it,' he once said. I think he rather liked the fact that I worked, and kept a photo of me half-naked on his phone to show his colleagues. I was a bit embarrassed.

'Darling, please tell them I am a writer too,' I said to him. I'd only been Samantha less than two years but I'd been a journalist almost 20. There was so much more to me than my sex work. I'd known and done more in my life.

But like all my relationships, it came to an end. His demise? He made the fateful error of recording the soccer on my Foxtel IQ. 'What the fuck?' I whispered when I scrolled down the recordings. '*Modern Family* as well?'

Other women would be secretly delighted – they'd see this as a sign he was keen, serious and he felt comfortable. Not me. Though I longed to be protected, the dullness of everyday life, of comfort and routine, annoyed me. I have no idea why. The poor sod watched *Modern Family* and soccer at my home all the time. But his recording of them betrayed his assumption that he was part of my future, and that I took offence to. It made me feel uneasy.

After painstakingly deleting every single episode I slammed down the controls, fuming.

'I want my key back,' I told him curtly. 'You're trying to take over. I don't want this.' I knew I was hurting him. After all, I'd given him the right signals. He cooked me dinner in my own home most evenings, and even met Luke to assure him that he wasn't out to replace him as Dad. On top of everything, his profession was perfect for my hypochondriac tendencies (I'd always secretly wanted my own personal doctor). Yep, my paramedic was a great catch.

But as soon as I felt a trickle of contentment, that niggling of comfortable coupledom, that was it. I was off. Full stop, end of sentence, next please!

No, that wasn't me. Give me loneliness any day. It's a feeling I can relate to, a feeling I am safe with. I love my own company. I find it hard to be vulnerable; to let someone inside.

After we ended things, I became mildly obsessed with someone far more suitable: a married client. He was a bigshot banker who took me on a business trip to Mexico. We did make the perfect couple, I convinced myself. We drank cocktails by the pool, shared tacos and walked on a beach in the evening. It was such a romantic time, marred only by his hiding behind rocks every few hours to call his young wife who had just given birth to their third baby. I know. Sounds pretty awful, doesn't it? But by now I was desensitised to marriage. Married, cheating men were a part of my regular working life.

One night while I was waiting for my client to finish a phone call, I met Anthony, a very loud but charming South African. The following day, while my client was out with business colleagues, Anthony and I spent eight flirtatious hours together at the bar. Months later, when I was back in Sydney, we continued to Skype each other, sometimes three times a day, declaring our undying love for each other. Anthony wanted to move countries and set up house with me. This felt like an unrealistic, unachievable love. To me, it was perfect.

Nothing physical happened between us, not even a kiss, but I liked him. He had huge, protective arms that I could imagine wrapping around me, shielding me from the world.

I even booked a ticket to visit him in Cape Town, but seven days before I was due to fly out, the reality of having something serious kicked in and, in true Amanda style, I cancelled.

'I'm really sorry, Ant,' I said late one night over Skype. 'But I can't come. I just don't want to now. I don't want to talk about it, but my mind is made up.'

He looked crestfallen. His kind eyes crumpled. Didn't he realise I did this kind of thing all the time? He suddenly seemed like a newbie at the whole relationship/fling thing. I stared at him, wishing I could feel something; sadness, regret, guilt. But pushing away was what I did well.

'You're blaady joking,' he said, in that accent that now grated on me. This poor guy had invested a fortune on me so far. He'd bought a Michael Kors handbag, new sheets for his bed, booked a safari and he even upgraded his Audi. He'd gone to the effort of telling his conservative family about the woman he met in Sydney, and I'd been invited to a family wedding. My name was on the table already. He even knew what I did and was okay with it (even though he'd told me, 'You won't need to do it when I am supporting you.').

'I'm sorry,' I said coldly, pressing the 'End Call' button. I might have even cried, but I couldn't deny the relief inside me, either. I didn't give a shit about the $2700 I'd lost on the plane ticket. That was two days' work for me.

I was alone and safe again. My best friend Tab once pointed out my bedroom had very bad Feng Sui for meeting someone. 'You need two of everything to open yourself up for love,' she remarked, as she climbed into my bed for a sleepover. 'Two tables, two lights, two cushions. You'll never meet anyone with just one of each!'

Oh really? So the next day, after she left, I heaved, pushed and finally managed to move my bed so it was squashed along the wall. Now it was impossible for anyone to climb in. I was cocooned in my solitary safe little haven.

No, I wasn't good at this thing called love. This thing people did, being part of a couple. Jesus, I saw enough and heard enough to put me off relationships for a lifetime. Being alone seemed a much safer place. Relationships were getting harder (not that I was much good at them before).

It was easier to disconnect at work; I'd been a working girl for two years now but that made it hard to rewire myself and feel real affection for someone else in my real life. The sex with the men I dated was always good, but that was Samantha. I could perform. I could make men happy in bed, no matter who I was that day. But what was I getting from it? Some kind of power trip? A little part of me secretly wanted a bit more. I knew I was sexy. But was I worthy of love? Did men not take me seriously when they knew what my job was? Was I trying to sabotage relationships by telling them I was a hooker – under this holier-than-thou guise of 'speaking the truth', or had I always been crap at relationships? After all, my ex-husband was a good and kind man. We lived in a lovely home, making family albums of happy events in our lives – engagement, babies – but it was too comfortable for me. Too conventional. Too forever. Is that why I just had to leave and become a hooker instead?

I came from a good family and went to a good school. But my younger years were spent living in terror of my mother's moods. When I left home at 18, I was never really allowed to return. I spent uni holidays sleeping on friends' floors, so stability was alien to me.

I remember Nina telling me that in her 12 years as a madam, all the sex workers she'd known had one thing in common: terrible relationships with their mothers.

'Everyone assumes you girls have daddy issues,' she remarked, 'but it's your mothers you don't get on with. Not having a solid female role model or something like that.'

I brought it up at The Bordello too. 'Who here has a crap relationship with their mum?' I asked on a quiet Sunday afternoon.

One hand went up, then another, then a sea of painted nails were raised in front of me. We looked around the room, half-laughing, half-shocked.

My mother and I love each other, but our relationship was at best strained. I always had the feeling she didn't really like me as a person. I think I pushed her buttons. If I walked into the room, she would quite often walk out. I tried hard to please her, but nothing was ever good enough. Christmas presents I carefully chose for her as a child were received coldly with the words, 'Did you keep the receipt?' before being stuffed in the back of her wardrobe and never used. I don't want to sound like I'm strumming the violins, but I can't pretend it wasn't hurtful.

I learnt at a young age the disconnection that would later come in handy as a sex worker. But I often wondered whether Samantha (whom I loved dearly) was wrecking my chance of finding love in the real world. Was she the real cause of my disconnection?

Maybe the client–worker relationship was all I needed, wanted and was capable of. It was certainly one I enjoyed. My needs were being met just as much as my clients' in our bookings.

A bit of a chat, sex, a cuddle, me thinking how lovely they are as I breathe in the final few wafts of their fragrance, while they probably think either 'God, she's a bit weird,' or 'she's lovely', or more likely, 'I reckon I've got one last go in me', and that is as complicated as it ever got.

Clients didn't fall in love with me. They may have got slightly obsessed with my breasts. They may have enjoyed talking to me. But men are kings of disconnection aren't they? Sure, I probably fell in love with a few (a lot actually) during our time together. Or at least, I certainly pretended to. But the truth was, I did have feelings for my clients. I liked them all, a lot. Because I knew our time would end. As soon as the buzzer went and I had walked them downstairs that fuzzy feeling evaporated – quickly replaced with 'who's next?'

It was a bit like speed-dating – but without the bullshit.

SAMANTHA
Tick tock

So here I was, established as Samantha at The Bordello. I wouldn't say I was running the show, but I was certainly one of their top girls – and I loved it. It was exciting. It was fun. One day I would be gulping back champagne with two other girls and two men in a dim, decadent room, dancing in a G-string, the next I would be perched on the end of a bed, handing a man a tissue and listening to how his wife treats him like he is invisible.

I loved the variety, the drama, the reality show. It was compelling. The night-shift girls would come in wearing pink Juicy tracksuits, Louis Vuitton bags and ugg boots, while the day girls arrived wearing summer dresses or jeans, flat shoes and always big sunglasses. The sort of woman you would pass on the street and admire her style. The girls at The Bordello were attractive, don't get me wrong; some were beautiful. They all had something special about them. But mostly they were your typical girl-next-door type: friendly, funny and pretty.

We came from all walks of life and careers: law, teaching, medicine, student, and so on. We came from different countries, too. The one thing we had in common was that none of us saw anything wrong with selling sex to men (in secret). Neither did we allow our work to take over our entire identity. We were mothers too, sometimes wives or girlfriends. But we were happy. Some of us had also given up our careers to do it. There were plenty of women, who, like me, had started out doing one or two days a week, dipping our (pedicured, Shellac) toes in. Once we realised it was actually fun and well-paid – bang. There went the day job.

Like I said, there was always a lot of laughter radiating from the changing room . . .

'So I went on a date with this hot guy, right, but I think I've fucked it up. We went for dinner, then back to my place. I put the condom on with my mouth, I jumped into all sorts of porn-star positions and afterwards, I passed him a drink and asked him would he like a massage with that. Do you think he might suspect I'm a hooker?'

This is the story told to me by the African girl from Adelaide who ditched her legal job because she was sick of the racism and decided to be a call girl instead. We were in hysterics. The poor guy either thought he'd hit the jackpot, or ran the other direction with his trousers still half done up.

I kept an eye and ear out for what management were up to as well. The office door was mostly closed. There was always lots of whispering come from the room, lots of decisions being made in there. Decisions such as who should be sent to our regular addict in the north coast, or which girl would be best for the businessman from Japan.

I'd drive home buzzing from all the gossip and drama, thinking that I could put together a TV show purely based on the goings-on in one day. But this time, I wasn't a lowly, badly paid writer getting off on some exclusive I was about to uncover. I was part of the show. No, scrap that. I was the *star* of the show. Every booking for me was like a miniseries. No matter how boring a client looked, he always had something interesting to say. The script would write itself. I could never shake the feeling that if only all women heard what I was hearing these men say, it would change so much. They would get it. They would get *men*.

I couldn't imagine a better way to earn money. I got to have sex all day! I got to work when I wanted! I was well and truly hooked.

I know this is the sex industry we are talking about. I know a lot of seedy stuff goes on. There are thousands of women working against their will in dingy depressing suburbs out there. I know that as I write this, there's a worker somewhere being abused by a client who thinks he has the right. But The Bordello was a far cry from that world. It was legal. As I've already made clear, I disagree with the notion that all sex workers are filled with self-loathing and rotten self-esteem. My confidence soared when I became Samantha. I agree that you need to be a certain type of personality to do this work. You need to be able to separate sex and love. You need to be able to see sex as an action not necessarily tied to an emotion, and the tricky thing is actually being able to recognise that warm, fuzzy emotion when you meet someone in your real life, after being trained to turn it off during work. But believe me, there are worse places to work. Women here turned up on the doorstep in their best clothes, almost begging for a job. I've seen them being interviewed by Raquelle or Roxy in the office. These girls wear their best clothes, too much perfume, and are filled with hope and excitement in their heavily-kohled eyes. They are drawn to the money, the freedom and the reputation of The Bordello.

But it wasn't perfect. And here are a few things I didn't really like about The Bordello in no particular order:

1) Management was about as trustworthy as a sexually frustrated married man.
2) The shifts were way too long (noon – 10 pm. Really?) You had to stay for your whole shift. You weren't really allowed to leave to go home (unless you had a good excuse) and you certainly were not allowed to leave the building to buy a coffee, which pissed me off, especially after the coffee machine broke down and they never fixed it. (I secretly think management couldn't be arsed to let the girls come out and use it every five minutes and reserved it only for guests.)
3) The way Raquelle would make passive-aggressive comments to girls. 'You look so pretty when you're wasted, Maggie,' I overheard her snipe to some girl late at night once. What was her problem? Was she jealous? I couldn't work it out.
4) Like at any job, there are bad eggs. In my case, there weren't bad eggs, just cracked ones. One girl decided to start bitching about me, saying I was sleeping with the owner (I wasn't), and that I was stealing clients and charging $100 for natural sex (as if). Like I needed more complications in my life.

5) The constant threat of being fired. I've got to hand it to management; they really made you feel you were working in the best place in the world and they always reminded you there was someone prettier waiting to take your place. Taking a client's number? Fired. Putting on too much weight? See ya.

I could go on, but I can't stand a whinger. Besides, I was making great cash and meeting great men and spending the days I wanted at home with my kids. But something started to happen. I started to get sick to death of my real job.

By this stage, I'd bagged one of the most sought-after roles in magazines. But my heart wasn't in it. I found myself staring out of the window of my grey office block at the five-star hotels, wishing I was there with a client instead. While I liked my colleagues, I started to disengage. I could no longer relate to – or enjoy – Friday night drinks or the office Christmas party. Not work the Friday before Christmas? That was at least $2000 I would miss out on. I noticed I was sensitive when people joked about 'hookers'. I had to bite my lip. Jesus, if only they knew.

The banalities of office life started to irritate me. Getting approval for a few days off? I had children, for Christ's sake. I didn't see them all the time. I wasn't going to let anyone tell me whether I could spend time with them or not. The most seductive thing about Samantha's job was not the money but the flexibility. Although I had Raquelle and Roxy to answer to, I was my own boss. If I didn't want to work all week, that was my decision. There was no leave form. No approval to seek. I just said 'I'm off' and it was easy as that. And when you're a single mum with two kids you don't see every day, you don't take kindly to someone else controlling your time off. I felt too old to be bossed around. My priority wasn't getting to the top of the ladder, but being with my kids, having spare time to do things I enjoyed like coffee with friends, walking my dogs, without the pressure to be somewhere, do something, for someone else.

So I decided to quit the media. The career I had dreamt of ever since I was a little girl was fading in its glory. I did feel that the changing media landscape meant journalism had shifted in a direction I no longer enjoyed, nor really wanted to be part of. News was no longer breaking in newspapers or TV but on Facebook and Twitter. It annoyed the crap out of me. Where was the skill in writing about some Hollywood celebrity? There were no qualifications needed to start a blog. Where was the actual journalism?

'I'm going freelance,' I whispered, not daring to look any of my colleagues in the eye.

And naturally, just as I decided to take the plunge, something very bad happened at work. It was my first real experience of the nasty side of my job and while it didn't happen to me, it affected me.

Let's call this man D. He worked in the fitness industry, but he never seemed to actually work: he was *always* at The Bordello, and not just for hour-long sessions, but for ten, sometimes up to 14 hours at a time. That was over $5000 a visit. He brought coke. He brought his laptop. And he brought his sick, sick fantasies.

He wasn't bad-looking, and he was tall and fit too, so when he picked me, I wasn't repulsed.

'One hour in room 3 please,' I said to Tiffany, handing her his black credit card, knowing, from what the girls had told me, he would keep on extending.

'Hey, you're okay with D?' she replied, looking at me.

'What do you mean?

'I mean, are you okay with D? You've seen him before right?'

'No . . .?'

Tiffany gave me a concerned look.

'Well, he's weird. The girls hate him. We hate him. But he spends a lot of money here. You don't have to see him, do you understand? You can say no.'

'Tiff, just fucking tell me will you?'

'Okay.' She inhaled slowly. 'He likes to talk. He's a talker. We think he's bisexual, but he has these fantasies . . .'

'Yes?'

'Of kids, all right? He gets off on talking about kids. But it's all talk. We don't actually think he does it in real life. Kids and dogs.'

I felt sick. So they did exist, these kinds of men, and they came to these places.

'I can handle him,' I said with an air of self-assured authority. Surely me, of all people, could handle this creep. I'd interviewed murderers. I'd had criminals justify to me why they did it. This loser? Easy.

And part of me was intrigued, too. It was the kind of compulsion we feel when we stop to look at an accident scene. Desperately craning our necks to catch a glimpse of a twisted foot or blood oozing onto the tarmac . . . *Oh, isn't that awful . . .*

Well, I wanted to see what this man had. I wanted to see what repulsion looked like.

Tiff was spot on. One second, this twisted little turd was panting on about some guy who lived in his apartment block, next he was telling me how he would love to fuck a German Shepherd. There was no sex. He wanted me to talk dirty while he masturbated. 'Oh, darling,' I breathed into his ear as he stroked his dick furiously. 'I've got the biggest Rottweiler at home that just loves her nipples being sucked.'

My poor dog. I winced internally as I said those words. I did have a Rottweiler at home and she would KILL me for using her in this sick fantasy.

Then D went onto his next subject. A boy he knew, who was nine. 'He is just so good-looking for a little kid,' he said quietly, testing the water, trying to look me in the eye.

'Of course he is,' I replied briskly, looking away, feeling my stomach turn with hate and fear, praying he was all talk. 'Young boys are so sweet.' I couldn't go there. I couldn't.

'You think I'm a paedo, don't you?' D replied, his eyes falling dark, his voice changing suddenly.

'No darling, I never said that,' I replied, choosing my words carefully, knowing D had a reputation for being volatile too.

'I'm really not. Here, look at my girlfriend,' he stammered, flicking through his photo album of his iPhone, showing me a smiling brunette. 'Why don't you give me your number? We can meet for a coffee . . . you're so beautiful . . .'

D was on edge. He darted from one subject to another, in between snorting line after line into his little piggy snout. Thankfully, there was no mention of children again. But as I walked out of that room, I decided D was right about something. I did think he was a paedophile.

And he proved himself to be one a few months later. It started off as a funny day – the sort of day when you feel something bad is going to happen, but you're not sure what. Like the sense of eerie calm just minutes before disaster strikes.

It was a Sunday. The Bordello was dead. There were hardly any girls on shift and the doorbell barely rang. Finally, I got a job. When I went to hand over the cash at reception, I noticed '12 hours' was on the computer screen in the King's Suite. 'Jesus!' I said to Tiffany behind the till. 'Who's in there?'

She looked sick. 'That disgusting man, D.'

'Who with?'

'Georgie.'

'The young one?' I replied. I was concerned now. Could she handle him for 12 hours? That was one hell of a headfuck.

The receptionist looked at me intently. It made me nervous. She was worried.

As soon as my booking was over, I scanned the girls' room. A forlorn figure dressed in a black trenchcoat was hunched over the bench. Georgie.

'Are you okay, George?' I said, cautiously sitting myself down next to her.

Silence. A sniff. A cough. She wiped her eyes and looked up.

'Not really.' And then she started crying. 'I saw . . . I saw . . . It was awful, Samantha, it was the worst thing I have ever seen.'

I swallowed, resisting the urge to talk. The golden rule as a journalist was that when someone was about to tell you something you absolutely need to know, you kept quiet. You didn't ask questions or butt in.

I put my hand on her shoulder and squeezed it. She turned away and blew her nose. Come on Georgie, tell me, I was thinking, Say it. SAY IT.

'I'm fine,' she whispered. 'I want to go home.' But I couldn't let this slip away. If D had been doing what I feared he had been doing, he couldn't get away with it.

'Georgie,' I said quietly. 'Did he show you pictures?' I said slowly. Georgie nodded, tears streaming now.

'Yes, Samantha,' she whispered, her voice breaking into a sob. 'He showed me pictures of children ... He showed me child pornography.' Her shoulders heaved. She was trying to contain, to mask any noise, as to not draw attention to herself.

I swallowed, closed my eyes. The sheer enormity of what I'd just heard, of what had been going on upstairs, made me feel sick. I'd heard lots of bad things, of course, as a reporter. But this felt somehow out of my league. I wasn't swimming with little fish any more. I was diving with Great Whites.

'Please don't say anything,' she whispered, getting up quickly and grabbing her bag. Was she scared she would lose her job? 'Just keep it to yourself. Please.'

I nodded. 'Of course, Georgie,' I lied, patting her back. 'I won't say anything to anyone, I promise.' Of course, I didn't mean a word of it. It was the only time, perhaps in my entire life, that I felt justified to lie. I waited until she had left the building before storming straight into the reception.

'Right,' I said, choking back tears. 'Where's D now?'

'Upstairs with another girl. Why?' replied one of the receptionists, barely looking up from her screen.

'That fucking disgusting prick showed Georgie child pornography and if you don't call the police, I will,' I said, trembling now. The receptionist went white and her mouth dropped opened, but no words came out. I ran to the bathroom and threw up.

What happened next was a blur of management shitting themselves and trying to do the right thing, but no one seemed to know what that was. They called Raquelle, who was on her day off. She called me from a crackly mobile to tell me she was coming in and for me to wait for her. D had left by now, back to his 'normal' life, taking his laptop of horror with him.

'Samantha, you have my word that I am equally disgusted by D's actions but we can't go around calling the police unless we have evidence,' Raquelle said in her patronisingly faux soothing voice, as she sat facing me, her large brown eyes flickering faster than usual.

But I wasn't going to be fobbed off here – not that I am saying that's what was happening. But here, in this world, we let things slide. What happened in The Bordello stayed at The Bordello. Men came here to cheat on their wives or girlfriends, or secretly indulge in their drug habits, and understood the discretion we offered. While we never, ever supplied drugs (and management sacked girls who were caught doing drugs), clients sneaked in their own stash. But this was different. It was a whole other deep, dark level.

'I understand, Raquelle,' I said curtly. 'But I was the one who spoke to Georgie afterwards. I know D's full name; I've seen his credit card. I have a duty of care not only to the girls who work here and as a mother, but also to children being abused. I don't care if I lose my job, but that man is going to be reported to the police even if I do it myself. I cannot sit back and do nothing. I cannot work in a place that turns a blind eye to child pornography.'

'And neither can I, Samantha,' Raquelle replied sadly, and I saw something I hadn't seen in her before: despair.

Raquelle looked pained. She looked panicked. And quite frankly, she looked out of her depth. What a pain in the arse for her that I was a fucking journalist. What a nosy trouble-maker I was that I had to probe into Georgie's tears, while most wouldn't, didn't, even notice the silent sobbing figure in the corner. And what a bloody thorn in her side that she knew I damn well I meant it when I said I was going to call the police. If she wanted to brush it under the carpet, she knew she couldn't.

In the end I didn't need to report him. Management did the right thing. I read in the papers a few months later that a male fitting D's description was arrested in the same part of town where he had once boasted to me about living (with his girlfriend, incidentally) and charged with possession of child pornography.

I emailed the link to Raquelle and I typed just two words. 'Got him.' She didn't reply. But she would have known this was a quiet victory. I'm not saying we busted a worldwide ring. Just one pathetic little man. I had no idea whether he was even charged in the end. But the shame, the mortification of having to explain his disgusting actions to his family, his colleagues, his girlfriend would have been crucifying for him. That in itself was extremely satisfying.

Although I didn't realise it at the time, this was the beginning of the end. Samantha's days at The Bordello were numbered.

Chapter Twelve

AMANDA

Revelations – and self-doubt

There is a horrid little man I see out and about. He sits around all day necking long blacks in a local café full of trendy-looking people, and trying to catch the eyes of pretty waitresses who serve him smiling, then roll their eyes when his back is turned. He clearly also scours the internet to pull a root (sorry – I meant pay for one as there is no way a girl would have sex with him for free). He somehow found a photo of me online at The Bordello website and has taken it upon himself to point out this amazing revelation to some of the local parents, one of whom asked me outright: 'Is it you?'

Oh for fuck's sake. 'Yes!' I replied in mock-horror. 'Yes it's me. I am an escort.' Woop de woo! There – the secret was out. The parent was shocked. 'Jesus,' he replied. 'I wouldn't ever admit that if I were you.'

Really? I wanted to say to him. *Really?* It was rich, particularly coming from him of all parents. This man, some big-time property developer, boozed it up on weekends and had told me how wasted he was going to get on the holidays. He'd told me about orders he'd put in for a pile of cocaine to stuff up his nose, about his dinner parties that ended up with mounds of white powder on mirrors as dessert. And he was a father. He'd be coming down from an illegal high when looking after his kids, but he was shocked at *my* behaviour? My legal job was somehow more worthy of his judgement than his own actions?

Even more frustrating was the fact that it was fine for the other loser to scour the net for sex, yet no one batted an eyelid. Because that's what men do, isn't it? But woe betide the woman who legally provides that service.

I don't have a drug problem. I've never had an addiction. I don't even smoke cigarettes. I hardly drink. Friends always get green tea when they drop in. Yet I'm the naughty one somehow, I'm the one breaking rules, the one who gets to be judged by people spending their weekends stuffing Class A drugs up their nose while their kids are asleep in Thomas the Tank Engine bed sheets?

For fuck's sake, this is 2014.

One guy I know started telling all and sundry he was 'shocked' I was a hooker.

'Dave S is telling everyone what you do,' my girlfriend told me over coffee one morning.

'Really? And how does Dave S know?' I asked.

'Steve told him.'

'And how does Steve know?'

'I dunno; you know how men gossip. They all talk.'

Oh God. Did I know how men gossip! Dave S was a regular at The Bordello. It was always the men (and usually the men who use sex workers) who had a problem with what I do, more so than women. Fear of getting busted, boys?

Let's get one thing clear. I didn't actually care what these people who didn't know me thought of me. Take the loser in the café who showed the dads my photos. It was mostly irritating. Even after I heard he was spreading rumours about me soliciting at the school gates, I had a good giggle. I don't think many fathers there can afford my rates these days.

These people have not much else going on in their lives so they like to gossip about and judge other people. Those who talk badly of others are actually showing their true colours. I think they must be unhappy, and while it annoys me, I also feel sorry for them. I don't have the time nor inclination to worry about what so-and-so is up to. If they're doing something naughty, good on them as long as they aren't hurting anyone.

What I care about are the people who know me and love me. My friends. They know me as Amanda. They know Samantha was always there, longing to escape the conventional life she was in. But they know me. They know I'm okay. They still throw their kids at mine for sleepovers. They still want to meet me for coffee. They still call me when they're upset. I am grateful for the friends in my life, because really, they are my family.

And most of the parents who know do not treat me any differently. They still call up wanting to have my children over for a playdate. My home is like a childcare centre most weekends, bustling with the kids playing guns and bouncing on our trampoline. Their parents know what I do for work and, except for trying to get me to tell them juicy stories, they don't act any differently towards me. If they were having a bit of a gossip behind closed doors, I wouldn't know: they don't say it to my face. And I'm thankful for that and lucky that I know nice, genuine people and I live in an eclectic, colourful community.

I know I am a good person. I know I am a good mother. My children are not just fed and watered. They are adored. Don't get me wrong: I don't spoil my children. I love them too much for that. But I am giving them the mother I always wished for myself, one who talks openly and candidly to them, even at their tiny young age; one who tells them how handsome and beautiful they are, how kind and sweet and funny they are, how clever they are. How they can be whatever they want to be, and be whoever they want to be, and most importantly, that they are beautiful *inside and out*. I make them look in the mirror and say 'I love you' to themselves. It sounds a bit hippie I know, but I learnt it from an expert. I am doing everything in my power to make my children feel they are adored unconditionally.

My children don't see me with men. They hardly see my boyfriends. They even pleaded with me to get a boyfriend once as 'Mummy you are always by yourself!' I rarely go out at night and leave them with a nanny. When I'm mum, I'm mum.

My profession has nothing to do with being a good mother, just like how any other job wouldn't define a person's parenting skills. Are neurosurgeons automatically awarded with 'Parent of the Year' certificates because of their job? If you are a banker, are you subsequently a good dad? If you are a teacher; does that make you a good mother? Do Catholic priests automatically make good people? Ha!

On the flipside, if you work in waste management, or don't earn a high income, would this make you a bad parent? I know a father who is a garbage collector, and he adores his kid more than life itself. He takes him surfing most afternoons and picks him up from school most days. His wife does odd jobs to pay the bills. Salt-of-the-earth folk and bloody good parents. Or there's the client I saw once, a gorgeous six-foot-tall hunk of a man. He was a criminal. I'm not talking petty crime here. But he had sole custody of his children. The judge decided he was a better father, despite his reputation (he had never been convicted of any crime). And I can believe that – he was a polite, respectful man. He spent the hour talking about how much love he had for those children of his. He even cut our hour short to go to Coles to buy food for their lunch the next day. He could teach a few dads a thing or two about fatherhood.

Okay, but here's a sticky issue. Would I want my daughter to do this job? Well, of course I bloody wouldn't. I wouldn't want her to try drugs, smoke cigarettes or have one-night stands either. I suffered from an eating disorder when I was a teenager and I would hate for my daughter to go through the agony of pinching her thighs every second of the day, counting each dimple of fat, or sleeping in pain because her bones jut out angrily.

My mother wasn't a hooker – far from it – and look how I turned out! Sex was disgusting in her opinion. If my kids are anything like any other children out there, they will want to be as different from their parents as possible. I'll probably get a daughter who will scold me when I am five minutes late, or refuse to pour me a second glass of wine, and choose the library over a night club any day.

But I do want my daughter to be empowered. I want her to come to me to talk about boys, sex and relationships. I respect myself, so I expect my daughter to respect me. I am not ashamed of who I am, and hopefully that will rub off on my kids. I want them to grow into open-minded and non-judgemental adults. I want them to accept people for who they are as a person, not what job they do, or what sexuality they are, or what the colour of their skin is.

Will my children approve of my job when they are older? Probably not. But they also wouldn't have approved of their father and I getting divorced. That didn't stop us. While I adore my kids, I am not going to live my life by what they would want. This is my life. I hope they will understand that Mummy did a funny job, but that Mummy was happy and she gave them the best life she could. She meant well.

I have a personality, rightly or wrongly, that can 'do' the sex industry. Whether it was my upbringing or whatever, I can do it; it feels easy to me. I see nothing wrong with helping humans feel a bit better about themselves. My work in tabloid journalism is what kept me up all night; not taking my clothes off in front of a man, not healing a troubled soul who was in need of some intimacy. I love what I do and I do what I love.

Am I responsible for the sexualisation of women? Well, it's not all my fault, is it! While I would love to claim responsibility for an issue in our society that has been going on for centuries, I can't take full credit for it.

One of my clients, a lovely gentle, kind man, used to be a drug dealer. He confessed to me as I was massaging his calf muscles. 'I never touched the stuff, but drug dealing set my family up. I bought a home, set up accounts for my kids, and then I got out,' he admitted. 'I'm not proud of what I did, but

I don't regret doing it. One day, when they're old enough, I will sit down and explain to them what I did and why I did it. I know more about drugs than anyone now. I can educate them on what drugs are made of and what they do to you. I believe in being honest with children. We underestimate their intelligence. Never be ashamed of who you are, as long as you are an honest person and a good person. Your children will love you for that.'

His words stuck. They came at a time when I was feeling insecure and ashamed of my job and terribly unsure as to whether to write this book. I spent many sleepless nights worrying about what so-and-so would think. I grilled anyone who would listen about what they thought; especially a few of my clients. Yes, me, the same person who didn't give a toss what people said behind her back when it came to the job itself.

Someone recently told me: 'Listen, darling: we both fuck people for money. At least you're honest about it.' He is an extremely successful banker in the city.

I thank my clients for their wise words, however difficult they were to hear at times.

We live in a society where kids have gay dads or lesbian mums. Where their mother may be black and they are white. Where, sadly, violence and sex are shown all too readily on TV and video games. America has a black president. We've been to the moon, old news. I read somewhere there will soon be hotels on Mars (Branson, where are you?). We have robots to do our washing up, aeroplanes with spas on board. Have we really not moved forward in our archaic attitude to the sex industry?

Would society rather I had a drinking problem and abused my children after a bottle of wine? Or how about a more normal situation, where I was absent at home, or at least mostly distracted, because I was having affairs? Or that the fights between my husband and I were keeping my kids up at night? Is that socially easier to swallow?

That said, I'm not being entirely fair. Every single person whom I have told about Samantha has been fantastic. While they may not show me their disapproval (if they do indeed have any), they have been extremely supportive and fascinated. Sure my life choice is not for them, but it doesn't mean that they no longer want me in their lives.

I ended up needing a nanny recently and confessed to her what I did. 'So, Bernice, if you have a problem with me working as an escort I suggest you look elsewhere for a job.'

'Amanda, darling,' she replied, patting my arm. 'I would have more of an issue if you worked for a tobacco company. What you do is fine with me.'

I've become a bit of a go-to for peoples' sexual confessions now. Maybe they think I am somehow an expert, that I have all the answers (I don't). But I am a good listener, and I don't judge.

Women whisper their sexual secrets to me and men open their hearts. They know I won't recoil in disgust or shock. Most men confess they have been to a sex worker, and I am beginning to see it is something 90 per cent of men do or have done, but they don't really talk about it with each other. Men tell me their wives or girlfriends always ask if they have been to a brothel or prostitute – and of course, they mostly lie. What's the point when it could be thrown back in your face for the next 20 years?

A married man I know confessed to me once he has a little rule for himself. If he is away on business, he treats himself to a girl. If he is really hungover, he will treat himself to a massage with a happy ending. 'I just tell the wife I'm going to Bunnings,' he grinned.

This man is happily married with young kids. His wife is sexy and gorgeous. Jesus, he would have been the last person I thought who would do it. But there you go.

Is what he does wrong?

I had an American client once who visited me three times in just as many weeks. A nice man, youngish, with sad brown eyes, broad shoulders and a shaved head. We never had sex. I just massaged him and listened to him talk about his life. 'Hey, I have a question. Should I be unhappy in a marriage, all the time?' he asked me on our first meeting. 'Is it supposed to be hard every single day?'

No, of course not. As he told me more, I could tell he wasn't in love anymore, but it was guilt and the kids that were making him stay. When he asked my advice, I sort of told him that too. But I wondered whether it was right for me to say so. Had I said too much?

I think it was the advice he really wanted. 'Hey, so is it right for her to want separate bedrooms?' he asked. 'She told me she's not attracted to me any more; what do you think?'

'I think you have a right to be happy,' I told him, kissing the back of his neck. 'Whatever that may be.'

Of course, I have no idea what her side of the story was, and I am sure she had a strong case too. But I knew her girlfriends would be taking care of her. They were her support network; I was his.

This client came back again one last time, a few weeks later. He paid for the hour, but sat on the bed still wearing his jeans. This time he was smiling.

'I can't stay today, Samantha,' he said. 'But I just came to say thank you. You won't see me again. But I wanted to thank you for helping me realise my marriage was over.'

He got up, kissed my forehead and left, closing the door gently behind him. It was hard to describe how I felt. A surge of self-satisfaction? Yes. Sad? He was such a nice guy and I knew he was on the right path now. But I also felt a sense of loss, knowing I would never see him again.

I thought about his wife. Great, so he made his mind up. But what about her? What do women do to 'let off steam' and get a release? Is it spas, health retreats and shopping trips? Where do we get our answers, our moment of clarity? Are we satisfied in our sex lives? If there was a bordello for women, would we go? Should we go? What kind of service would we want? I always say for every husband that comes to The Bordello, there's an unhappy wife at home.

To every single one of us who thumbed *Fifty Shades of Grey*, what were we searching for? Excitement? Illicit sex? While our husbands are out to play, how do we get our thrills?

I've already told you that I think I save some marriages. Part of what I do is give husbands some form of release. They come, they cum, and they go back happy husbands.

Is that cheating? Is it wrong? Hey don't shoot me! I'm the mere messenger (sort of). Would you really divorce your husband because of that? Most men I meet don't want affairs. They don't want the hassle and headache of two women. Their lives are busy enough. They just want to see and feel another naked body sometimes.

Of course, being Samantha, I should say no. Of course it's not wrong! Of course men and women should be allowed to sleep with whomever they want to sleep with. It's just sex, after all.

I used to believe that, and maybe I still want to. But the longer I spent working as Samantha, the more traditional

I was becoming. I stopped having sex in my real life. I stopped dating. I'd had enough of meaningless encounters. I wanted to believe in true love, I wanted to believe it could happen. Would I want the man I love touching, feeling, stroking another woman, regardless of whether there was a wad of cash in a white envelope next to the bed?

Love needs boundaries. It needs trust. It needs commitment. Society needs rules.

While I would understand why he is doing it, how could I not feel jealous, insecure and pissed off?

No, I wouldn't be too happy about it. I may understand men but I don't always agree with them.

SAMANTHA
The patient

Men always disrupt good daytime telly watching.

'Sammy, you've got a client waiting for you,' Roxy yelled out from the doorway of the changing room.

I rolled my eyes. They certainly know how to ruin my good time. Why did I have to get called up now, when I was sitting on a sofa, in stockings and a suspender belt, my feet on the coffee table, eating pasta and watching *Dr Oz*?

'Okay,' I sighed, slamming down my fork. I wasn't in the mood for this today. I didn't want anyone touching me, I didn't want to make conversation while massaging a hairy back. I wanted my lunch and a bit of trashy telly.

'Hello, darling,' I sang as I threw open the door. Who was this little annoying twerp who had ruined my lunchtime break?

'Samantha,' he said, looking up, his eyes hopeful. 'It's Brett. Do you remember me?'

I blinked. Yes I did remember him. He was a sweet man, young, tall, handsome with a gap in his teeth, big wide forehead and kind eyes. A single dad, whose marriage broke down after his son passed away, though he still had three other children he shared with his ex-wife. Impressed that I remember their story? A good journalist, or sex worker, never forgets.

But something was different. I glanced down and noticed a long transparent tube angrily protruding from his arm. There was a white bracelet on his wrist with his name and his date of birth. Hang on . . .?

'What's wrong with you?' I said, linking his arm as we walked upstairs. 'What's all this?'

'I'm in hospital. I discharged myself to come and see you,' he said, pulling out his wallet. 'I'm not good, Samantha. It's my heart. They're worried about me.'

Without going into too much detail, Brett had an inherited heart condition from birth. He was well when we had met before, but now a severe infection meant he was tied to a hospital bed. He'd just spent ten weeks in intensive care and though he was on the mend, doctors were concerned the infection might come back.

'It was touch and go at one stage,' he said quietly, struggling to take his shoes off. 'I'm in there for another few months at least. But I had to come and see you Samantha, I just had to.'

The concern on my face turned to a smile. Of course he had to – a man going without sex despite almost dying? Unheard of! Flattering – and dramatic. Did he rip off the cords from his IV drip and stagger across the freeway to find me? Has he left the doctors baffled as why his bed is mysteriously empty? 'I might even go to Hungry Jack's after this,' he smiled, pulling me close. 'Now come here, sexy . . .'

I breathed in the scent from his neck – he smelt sterile, of chemicals, the unloving soap you get at hospitals. It made me feel sick, but I buried that away. I liked Brett; he was a good man. He wasn't wealthy, or a major success in life. But he was honest and reminded me of one of my ex-boyfriends in London. The sex was awkward but loving in a funny way if you know what I mean. The tubes were hardly a turn on, and I was worried I was going to hurt Brett. He wanted to spend most of the hour hugging me and breathing in my hair. It made me sad to see someone who was so fit and so good-looking turn into a fragile shell.

I didn't know what I found more shocking. The fact that he'd nearly died, or the fact that he'd discharged himself to come and see me, with his tubes and wires still poking out of his body. I watched him as he shuffled around the room sadly. Poor Brett, I felt terrible taking his money. He had gone through enough losing a child, a marriage and now his health. And he wasn't even 30. Sometimes, life just wasn't fair.

I often wonder about Brett. It was just another close encounter with a stranger, really, whom I grew to like and probably will never see again. But I was beginning to get too close to my subjects. And good journalists and sex workers can't afford to do that.

Chapter Thirteen

AMANDA

Whore or a thief?

The beauty of coming from Europe is that I always have somewhere nice to go to on holiday. True, it may be my parents' house, with evenings spent watching reruns of *Only Fools and Horses* as opposed to propping up at a sophisticated bar with some bubbles. But it's in a jolly nice area and the kids love it.

It does mean three weeks of mounting tension for my mother and I, which invariably ends up in a screaming, scathing row, but it's nothing I have not prepared myself for. A bit like a hurricane warning: you know it's coming, you prepare the best you can and hope you survive. You batten down the hatches and pray it ends soon with little destruction.

I don't dislike my mother. I love her and I know she loves me. I feel awful writing these words, but I am a teller of the truth, and this is the truth. Even she can't deny our relationship has always been strained. The tension between us would be equal to a Valentine's Day dinner with a couple where the wife has just found out her husband had visited me.

Last year, I took the kids for three glorious weeks to Europe. Roxy knew Samantha was on leave and the clients could wait. The trip was good; bearable. Once the predicted fight with my mother was over, which resulted in my going to bed crying, and her coming up with two glasses of red to apologise, the tension eased.

I left a few weeks later feeling happy and satisfied that my parents had spent a few good weeks with their grandchildren. Holiday tick, now back to work.

Did I tell my parents about my new career? Of course not. I was tempted to confess all, especially after a few glasses of rosé, but some things are best left unsaid.

Until I got the phone call from my sister, once back in Sydney.

'Mum thinks you've taken her gold rings.'

'What?'

'Mum thinks you took her jewellery when you were out there.'

'Sorry – she *what*?' I wasn't making sense of this conversation; the words too obscure for me to comprehend.

'Remember when Mum showed you all her jewellery on her bed?'

'Yeah?'

'Two of her gold rings are missing and she thinks you've taken them. I know it's stupid, please don't get upset Amanda.'

I slammed the phone down with tears stinging my eyes. For Christ's sake. Did my mother really think her own daughter would steal from her?

When my four-year-old found \$10 on the pavement, I insisted we go to Vinnies and spend it. 'We need to give it back to the poor children, darling,' I said. But I don't need to justify myself. If you've read this far, you would have worked out that you could call me many things, but a liar and a thief I am not.

I texted my father. 'What is Mum's problem with me?'

He texted back: 'I know Amanda, sorry. Tried sticking up for you.'

Useless. I was a 39-year-old woman, and still being reduced to a quivering mess by my mother. The hurt and the pain was like nothing I had felt before. I could handle rude clients, people calling me old or too fat or too skinny, and I could handle being dumped. But being accused of stealing by my own mother, no, I couldn't get over this. I couldn't brush this under the carpet.

When Dad eventually called me, it was only in secret. My mother had told him not to speak to me.

'I know, love,' he said in a hushed tone. 'It must be very hurtful. Of course you didn't take her rings. I tried to persuade her . . .'

'Why, Dad?' I said, tearfully. 'Why me? What has been her problem with me? Why does she hate me?'

'She doesn't hate you,' he replied, trying to comfort me. 'But I suppose she has never really liked you.' He laughed nervously, probably hoping I would take his words as lightly as he said them.

Like little bullets, those words tore through my heart. Wow. Now even I had to hand it to him; that was painful. Was I really that unlikeable?

I didn't want to make Dad upset. It wasn't his fault. 'Okay, thanks Dad,' I mumbled, hot tears falling onto my phone. 'Speak later.'

My grief turned to anger pretty soon. Fucking useless, the pair of them, I thought furiously. I was sick to death of this. Dad wasn't allowed to call me; Mum thought I was a thief. I mean, could they really think any less of me? And did I really care anymore?

At home that evening, while brushing my daughter's hair and helping my boy with his Lego, the tears came. I adore my children. How could a mother not LIKE her child?

As parents, aren't we supposed to nurture our kids as best we can? Are we supposed to love them unconditionally?

The constant stream of pain I had to endure from an ocean away was from my family. I was over this. Not only did I not want to expose myself to their toxicity any more, but also did not want to risk exposing my children to it.

So I wrote the email. THAT email. The one that told them I am an escort. That I was safe and happy, but that I could no longer deceive them and no longer be ashamed of who I am. That I actually liked who I was, even if she didn't. That, quite frankly, I would rather be called a whore than a thief, and that sorry Mother, but I could no longer have a relationship with someone who thought I was capable of stealing. 'I've lost one parent this week, I am prepared to lose another,' I punched out on the laptop. Send.

Shit.

A few emails flew back and forth. Anger, hurt, dismay (from them). Anger, hurt, dismay (from me).

That was months ago. We haven't spoken since. My 40th came and went; nothing. Not even a card. I got sick with pneumonia, probably due to stress. My phone remained angrily silent.

Of course it's upsetting. I feel lost without them, even if they were at best clipped tones on the other side of the world. I still and always will love them.

But I'm not sorry. I am not apologising for who I am, because it doesn't sit well with them. I am not sorry for being honest.

I'm sad my parents are missing out on their only grand-children. I'm sad that Christmas was gifts in the mail for my kids, but no phone call. I'm sad because I know they will be sad. But I am not sorry. I've always pretty much been alone, and I am alone now. It's something I am used to.

For the first time in my life, I stood up to my mother and I felt good. They had left me no choice. I think Samantha's confidence was filtering through to other parts of my life and having a good influence, believe it or not. I'm not sure I would have had the nerve to stand my ground if Samantha wasn't there, her hand on my shoulder, urging me to show strength.

Would my parents prefer me to live a lie? Would they prefer to never know their daughter? It certainly seems that way. That's not me. I am not going to change who I am in case it upsets people, or ruffles a few feathers. If you don't like me, or don't approve of my life, don't be in it. Fuck off.

My parents made their choice and I respect them for that.

Telling my family empowered me. There's that word again: empowerment. Feeling of power from within. A feeling I was used to having these days and a feeling that was soon, unbe-known to me, going to be taken away from under my nose.

SAMANTHA
The smiling psychopath

God I loved this job! That man, the good-looking one in the meeting room, with a blue-and-white checked shirt, blue sparkly eyes and sexy smile, he picked me! I knew he would. The minute I waltzed in, he looked up and his face brightened. 'Wow,' he exclaimed, trying to grab my hand. 'Come and sit down.'

I met his gaze and grinned. Hmm, dishy! There was something about that face. So cute, so familiar? 'Have I met you before?' I asked teasingly, but I meant it. I knew this face . . .

'No, I don't think so,' he replied, stroking my cheek. 'I'd remember it if I had.'

I kept on flirting but his face was bugging me. Those eyes, that smile? Now come on, Amanda, think. Where did I know him from? The café? The beach? Here? I usually was so good at remembering clients. Why couldn't I recall this one? *Flick*

flick flick went the memory bank in my head, but I couldn't find it. Not yet. I couldn't care that much, though. With his RM Williams boots, nice jeans and big strong hands, he was gorgeous!

We linked arms and I practically danced up those stairs.

'One hour, gorgeous,' he said, handing me the cash. 'But I'll probably stay a few more with you!'

As I walked to cashier, it was beginning to annoy me. I knew him, I did! 'Tiff,' I said handing over the money. 'Where do I know that man? The one in room 6. I know him.'

'Have you seen him before? He's a regular.'

'No, I don't think so.'

But this wasn't like me! Why couldn't I remember?

I poured him a vodka, and myself a gin, but I didn't touch mine. It wasn't even lunch-time; too early in the day. Maybe he was celebrating. 'Hey we don't know each other from the real world, do we?' I said, passing him his glass.

'No,' he replied, taking a few big slurps. He told me about his job; he owned a restaurant. He told me his name was T, that he lived in the inner city.

He had a quick shower while I made the bed, my mind still whirring.

'You're not married to a friend, are you?' I shouted out, half-joking.

'No, darling, I'm not. I wish I did know you in the outside world!' Then he came out of the shower and pulled me towards his wet body, kissing me firmly on the lips.

I looked up and smiled. But his eyes darkened. His facial expression darkened. 'Come here,' he growled, and he pulled me close. Then he threw me onto the bed and climbed on top, pinning my arms beside me. I froze.

And then I remembered. His kiss. I remembered. His pushing hands on my body. *I remembered.*

I knew this man. He had been a client a year ago. He was rough with me, too rough. I was too shy to tell him at the time, a bit shaken. His nice demeanour and good looks had thrown me. But I remembered his touch. I remembered his rough kiss.

'Look, T . . .' I said, pulling myself up. 'I remember you now. You are rough. I don't want you to be rough with me today, do you understand? If you are too rough with me, I will end this session and I will leave. Is that clear?'

'Shh,' he whispered, completely ignoring me. 'Besides, I never listen to what this says,' he said, pointing to my mouth. 'I listen to what *this* says.' And he moved his hand to my panties, tearing them off, before shoving his fingers inside.

'T, no,' I protested, trying to reach my hands up to push him away. But my body felt like wood; I couldn't move. I was paralysed, from shock more than fear. This wasn't really happening, was it?

It was.

'No,' I croaked as he pushed me around, hands, fingers inside me, deep, hurting me.

'It hurts T, stop, it really hurts,' I pleaded, but it was almost as if my pain was driving him even more.

There was no point in my protesting. I tried to cross my legs and struggle free; I tried to protest and push him off. But he was strong and defiant.

The assault lasted an hour. In that time, I had said no probably 30 times and tried to wriggle free, only to be pinned down, with T just smiling at me, whispering, 'Shh.'

In the end, he threw my face in the pillow. I felt him inside me. 'No, T,' I pleaded again. 'Not without a condom.'

Too late. He won.

Why didn't I get up, run out, or press the buzzer? Because there was a part of me that thought he was going to stop. But he never did.

I was frozen in shock. Had I been too friendly? Too smiley? My mind replayed the scene as he was on top of me, grinning, hurting me.

Afterwards, bruised and sore, I got up. 'T, you've just raped me,' I said quietly, pulling a towel over me.

'Ahh,' he replied in mock sympathy. 'Let's extend an hour and I'll give you a massage as redemption?'

I looked at his glass of vodka, the ice now melted. I resisted the urge to pick it up, smash it and hold it to his Adam's apple, stabbing at his skin until blood oozed out.

'You need to go,' I whispered. 'You need to go *now.*'

'Really? You don't want to extend?' he replied, looking at me confused. That threw me – did he not understand?

I showed him to the front door. Then I went to reception and told them what happened before bursting into tears. They were great, handed me tissues, rubbed my shoulders. But I was stoic, I'd be okay. I barely told anyone that day. It was just rough sex that went out of control. It was okay.

My next client was an angel in disguise. A heavy man, wearing a turban and a smile, paid for an hour. I poured myself a strong drink, and then another, then another. So many of my clients did this – could I? Numbing my feelings, blocking out the pain, the shame. I could do this. I could. It was just rough sex, a bad client. We've all had them.

But of course, I broke down. Before I even took my clothes off I started to cry. I stared at myself in the ice bucket, my face all red and puffy. 'I'm sorry – I'll make sure you get your money back,' I said quietly, blowing my nose. 'I just had a bad client, I'm sorry. It's not you.'

'Hey, don't worry about that, what did he do?' said this kind man, with concern on his face.

'He was just a bit rough with me and he didn't stop.' I choked up, trying to swallow the big painful lump in my throat. I was so ashamed I couldn't meet his eyes.

'Listen,' he said seriously. 'I want you to do something for me. I want you to go home tonight and look in the mirror. Look at yourself in the eyes and say "I'm a good person." Say it loud and say it ten times.'

His kindness made me cry more. This time, it was my turn to use the shoulder of another in these rooms. 'Thank you,' I said, smiling through my tears. 'What's your name?'

'Sunny,' he said. 'My friends call me Sunny because I am always happy.'

I went home and did what he said but looking back, I was on autopilot, still in a daze. Was it rape? Can a client rape a sex worker?

The next day, I told Raquelle. It just came out of my mouth as we were standing by the nut bowl. She asked me how my week had been as she dived her hand into the almonds.

'Not great,' I replied quietly, picking up an almond and studying it like it was suddenly the most fascinating nut I had ever seen. 'A client assaulted me.'

She took me into the office and made me tell her everything. How he pinned me down, he turned me over, threw my head in the pillow, and raped me without a condom.

'Samantha,' she said, visibly upset. 'That is not okay here. You call me if you need me, all right?'

I worked the next day but I drank a lot, which was so unlike me. Went home, passed out. The next day, work again. My first client spent two hours smoking ice in front of me as I watched. It was early on a Sunday morning. I just stared at the smoke curling up as he danced to the music alone, stared at myself in the mirror as I showered. Was this the beginning of my end? I loved this job so much. Samantha was the strong and courageous one out of us two. If she fell apart, what would happen to me?

The buzzer went, but I sat there, watching him dance. For a split second, I wanted to get high, to block the pain I was feeling, just like him. Drugs, though, were never my vice. T may have taken my power away, but he wasn't taking my sanity. He wasn't going to take my health.

I ended up going thirty minutes over time. 'Didn't you realise?' the receptionist snapped.

'Yeah, well, maybe don't put me in a room with a man smoking ice at 10 on a fucking Sunday morning,' I snapped back, before marching downstairs.

Moments later, Raquelle took me aside. 'You need to take some time off,' she said firmly, her hand on my shoulder. 'You need to leave now. Call a sexual assault counsellor, call someone. But you can't be here any more until you have some time off.'

'Raquelle, I'm fine,' I interrupted, upset now and trying to fight back tears. 'I've got bookings and –'

'No, you're not fine and you need to take time off.' There was no point arguing with her. She was a manager and it was her call. She helped me open my locker and take my bag out, then she walked me out of the back door in silence. The other girls stared as she ushered me out.

'Goodbye, Samantha, take care of yourself,' she said, not meeting my eyes, and she closed the door behind her.

Little did I know that would be the last time I stepped in or out of The Bordello.

Chapter Fourteen

AMANDA
Dumped

So in the space of a week, I'd lost my parents and my job. Samantha had left the building and was never coming back.

Leaving the job wasn't my choice, of course. I might have been too naive to figure it out at the time, when Raquelle was escorting me out.

I didn't realise that not long after she closed the door behind me, my profile was deleted from the website, removing any trace of me. I had no idea that the emails and phone calls I made were going to be ignored.

Instead, I went home and sent this email. *'Hi Raquelle, I just wanted to say thank you for today. If you hadn't had a chat with me, I would have bottled it up and that wouldn't have been healthy. Thank you for encouraging me to seek help. I am blessed to work in such a professional establishment.'*

No response.

I called a few days later. 'Hi Tiff, it's Samantha. Can you ask Raquelle to call me back please?'

'No problem, Samantha,' she replied in a softer voice than usual. 'And listen, you take care okay? We miss you.'

But Raquelle didn't call back. Funny, when she wanted you to do something, to go and see a coked-up party boy in a hotel somewhere, she would be attached to her phone. But now, when she actually had to act like a professional? Nothing.

I was beginning to feel uneasy, and the assault was affecting me more than I wanted. I tried to perk myself up, went to the gym, smiled a lot, drank coffee in bookshops. But there was a heavy sadness inside me that I couldn't shake, and an annoyance that was growing. And now I might have lost my job, which was the biggest kick to my guts of all.

Who could I tell? Even though my friends knew what I did, I felt ashamed to tell them about this. I was afraid that by telling them I'd been raped at work I'd be confirming their worries. I was so pro the industry, pro sex work, pro female empowerment. All those critics in society telling me how dangerous it was, how disempowering it was – were they being proved right? Was Dan, the lovely cop, right?

And it made me angry. Really angry. The whole bloody point of being Samantha was that she was empowered. She was in control. That's why I steered away from drugs and drinking. If you lost control, you lost the game. Clear head, sharp mind. And I never lost control. I never gave up my power. But this man had managed to take it away from me. In just one hour, he did something that I could never, ever forgive him for: he killed Samantha.

But who could I tell? Who would listen? Raquelle had made her position clear, that was for sure. It wasn't going to be her. These were thoughts swirling around in my head one morning, as I was out walking. Past the shops, the cafés, and the police station . . . *the police station.*

'I would like to report an assault,' I whispered to the receptionist. Seconds later, in a room, with a box of tissues and a detective. I gave him a snapshot version of what happened, while he scribbled down some notes.

'Look, I am going to be straight with you, but you need to be straight with me,' I said bravely. 'I am a sex worker. I was raped by a client. If this is all going to be too hard and going to waste your time and my time, I would rather not go through it.'

'It's not going to waste our time,' he replied kindly. 'You're not just a sex worker. It's your word against his and from what you tell me, you have a very strong word.'

Just telling my story, having someone take it seriously, even just for an hour, I felt validated. I didn't want to be a victim. I wanted that man to pay – just like D the paedophile. I knew this would probably never get to court. But I wanted the burning humiliation of police turning up at his work and asking him questions. I wanted him to toss in bed wondering whether his career and life would be over.

A few days after that, I sent an email to work. *'Raquelle, just thought you should know I have notified the police. They are investigating now and probably will want CCTV footage. Sorry this is a pain. I'm ready to come back to work.'*

No response.

Bar turning up at the front door like a mad woman, I felt utterly lost and in despair, like being dumped for no reason by someone who wouldn't return my calls. Why wasn't she responding? I was at my lowest and needed a bit of support from her. I'd given that place a good year or so of my life, made them good money and had a great reputation there. Had I not earned some form of respect? I clicked onto the website and scanned the profiles and pictures of all the girls. I was usually just before Sarah and Savannah. There was nothing. I was gone. Samantha had been wiped off the face off the earth.

'Please, just call them,' I wailed to a male friend. 'Try to book me and see what they say.'

He called back minutes later. 'The woman said you've gone on holiday and are unlikely to return.'

I was devastated. I suppose it was a bit like finding out your husband was leaving you for another woman and he wasn't coming back. At first, disbelief. Then anger. And now, a slow realisation. The fucking bastards.

Samantha was no longer welcome at The Bordello because she got raped.

Or was it because I went to the cops? Were they worried because I used to be a reporter and they knew I was writing a book? Or because I was one of those women who always wanted to do the right thing and quite frankly, they didn't want girls like me, they wanted girls who kept their mouths shut.

Whatever their reason, I needed communication. Tell me it's over – don't cut me out. Do the right thing. Didn't I deserve that?

And this is how the sex industry sucks. In what other industry could you get fired and not KNOW you'd been fired? Where else could an assault on their premises cost you your job? No redundancy, no workers' rights, not even a box of chocolates and a We'll Miss You card. I had scoffed at friends worried about my 'safety' – yet they were proved right. I was supposed to be safe. I was supposed to be in control. I was supposed to be pro the sex industry. My faithful friend had let me down.

It was a terrible few weeks. The police weren't getting anywhere in their investigation. My hormones were going haywire and I put on a few kilos. I had a feeling my Mirena (IUD) had been dislodged in my assault, causing bloating and mood swings (just what I needed) and I was right. A check-up at the doctor and an ultrasound confirmed that yes, my coil had been 'misplaced' due to the rough nature of my perpetrator and I had to have it surgically removed and replaced. Not very nice.

The sexual assault counsellor was, in my opinion, useless. She was wearing tie-dyed trousers and a nose ring. Hippie scribes were on the wall, with an incense stick burning, taking me back to my depressing student days. For a second there, I was half-expecting her to get out some Tarot cards and start reading from them.

I couldn't help but feel she was quietly judging me as her eyes slowly flitted down from my chest to the shoes I was wearing (battered Nike runners).

'Hmm,' she nodded when I told her what happened.

'Ohh,' she said when I told her work hadn't called back.

'Mmm,' she said when I cried into my soggy tissues.

Luckily for me, my therapist Doris was amazing. A woman of my age, a mother and non-judgemental. She wouldn't just nod and wander off in her head about what she was having for dinner. We conversed, we laughed, she listened and I cried.

With Doris, Tab and a few other close friends around me, I felt supported and I felt loved. I booked myself for a health spa, but just before I went, I decided I wanted closure, clarity and comfort in my head. I wanted to make sure that I'd done the right thing. On Boxing Day, when the kids were at their dad's, and the dogs had polished off the turkey, I opened my laptop and wrote down the words that came into my head. There was no planning, no preparation, not even spellcheck.

And here it is, word for word.

Dear Raquelle,

Firstly, Merry Christmas. I sincerely hope you & the team are having a lovely break.

Secondly, judging by your silence and refusal to respond to my emails and calls, I am to presume I no longer have employment with The Bordello.

I am also to presume it is because I was raped on your premises, and probably because I reported it to the police.

I just wanted to say, as I am sure you know already, that your behaviour Raquelle, has been absolutely appalling. Seeing as you are a) an advocate of the sex industry and b) female, the way you have handled this has been truly unprofessional.

Your treatment of me was far, far worse than being raped. The rape itself was unpleasant, I had to have my Mirena surgically removed and a new one put in because he was so violent. That I can get over, but the shocking way a so-called professionally run brothel has treated the whole situation has been absolutely shameful, prehistoric and out-dated.

It is such a shame my time at The Bordello ended on such a sour note.

I am not expecting a response from you, however, as you know, I saw my job as a proper job, and I like to act always with honesty, professionalism and with integrity. I needed to have closure, which now I have.

Have a wonderful New Year and good luck in the future.
Amanda

I signed it with my real name because I wanted to show her I was not ashamed of who I was, like so many of the girls there. I was not afraid to give them my identity; she wasn't going to have any power over me. No one was.

Once again, I received no response. But I had expected that. For me, it meant closure. It was the end of 2013. It had been a terrible few months, losing my parents, now my job. Going to a health retreat was just what the doctor ordered. And there, in the rolling hills and serene setting in Queensland's hinterland, I got the solitude I needed. It gave me peace and calm in my whirring head. The only noise was the buzzy hum of cicadas at night and the rustle of grass, as wallabies foraged for food. There was no escaping my head here. There was no make-up to hide under, no stilettos to slip into. Samantha wasn't welcome here. Amanda had to do this one by herself; there was no hiding. It was, uncomfortable as I felt, just me, myself and I. But it was just what I needed. Being alone gave me the time and space to think about what my next move was going to be.

Had Samantha really died, or had she just gone on a much needed break? Did I really want to kill her off for good?

I didn't just take a few weeks off, I took a few months. Not at the health retreat of course – what a luxury that would have been! – but at home. When the kids were with their father, I pottered around the house. I rarely went out at night – instead I spent my time gardening, potting plants, watching new life grow. I spent lazy summer afternoons in my backyard drinking tea with good friends, walking the dogs and writing. Time to gather my clattery thoughts and put them in a box. Time to heal.

Amanda

I didn't realise it at the time, but I needed this break. The assault, my family – of course it was all going to affect me. It just took its time in doing so. I was so used to not feeling, not connecting, that finally, all the things I hadn't felt and connected with came pouring out. I'm not the crying type – I didn't spend days in bed with a box of tissues. That's not my style. I needed sunshine, not stale bed sheets; people, not solitude. Instead I poured my energy into being healthy, reconnecting with friends, cooking.

I kept replaying the scene with T in my head over and over again. What did I do wrong? What would I do next time? Would there ever be a next time? Was it my job that was dangerous or my lack of boundaries? My gut tells me it was the latter.

A girlfriend I worked with went to The Bordello and asked to empty my locker. 'How is Samantha?' Tiff asked her, handing her the key.

'She's fine,' replied my friend. 'But she isn't coming back.'

'Tell her we miss her and give her our love,' was Tiff's reply. I appreciated her words – my departure had nothing to do with the receptionists, who were all lovely, hardworking women.

It was funny, really, but of all the jobs I'd had, all the high-profile, highly sought after roles in the media, this was the job I was going to miss the most.

Despite it all, I had no regrets about Samantha and The Bordello. I worked there for the best part of 18 months. I made good friends whom I still speak to today. I met some lovely, lovely men, who helped me in their own little ways, helped me understand their sex and how their brains are wired (a lot differently from women's, but we knew that already!). I learnt a bit about marriage and relationships, and I witnessed some tragic men who were whirling in their own world of pain and used drugs and alcohol to numb their senses.

I am still trying to work out whether I was simply crazy to become a worker. Was I absolutely mad to be telling people? Would I look back on these years on my deathbed and wonder what the hell was I thinking?

But just as quickly, my thoughts turn to the men I've met and the issues we've talked about: their marriages, their loneliness, their inability to deal with those issues with anybody besides me.

As a society we prefer to brush these sticky issues under the carpet. We prefer to talk about the weather and how lovely our summer holiday was. We talk about happy events like engagements, marriages and kids. But scratch beneath the surface of any marriage and relationship and you'll find it – some bone of discontent. And then, bingo! You've hit 55 and you wonder why your marriage is so lonely. (I'm talking about men and women here).

The only people I need to justify my life choices to are my children, when the time for that conversation comes.

I learnt, believe it or not, that as women we should learn to love our bodies just as they are. When I say my confidence soared as Samantha, I wasn't joking. I stopped hating my thighs and bum, and I started to see what others saw in them. I realised that sexy meant confidence, not skinny legs. I learnt the most attractive thing about a woman was her smile. I actually learnt about boundaries. My experience with T taught me I hadn't finely tuned that bit. My shock at his treatment of me should have turned to strength, but it didn't. But you know what? It will next time, if it happens again. You don't need to be a sex worker to be assaulted – just read the papers.

I wasn't bitter that my time ended there so harshly. In fact, as the days passed, I became relieved. Maybe Raquelle knew my time was coming to an end and did me a favour. I like to think so. I look back now not in hate or anger but gratitude and understanding, and Raquelle, if you are reading this, you're a braver woman than me. Strong and confident as I am, I don't think I could do what you do. Your job isn't a kind one, no matter how you disguise it with smiles and pats on the back, sending bright-eyed girls off to strange hotel rooms with strange men.

I thought about going back to work, but I wasn't ready in any capacity. Samantha had been such a big part of Amanda's life, for the past 18 months or so since she was born, and I wasn't sure Amanda had really got much of a word in edgeways. It was all about Samantha. Her energy, her humour and her voraciousness. Amanda needed to come out of her shell a bit and let Samantha go. And as the weeks rolled by, and clarity slowly showed its face, I started to feel more grounded and connected. I even met a man (let's call him the boy with the dog) – walking our dogs on an inner-city beach. Now I had the time to spend with someone without having to rush off to my next shift, and it was nice. I cooked him dinners of meat and crispy rice, Middle Eastern style, and we would cosy up of an evening watching sport on TV (I do still like to accommodate men in some ways).

He knew about my past, and accepted it. 'Just don't ever lie to me,' he said over dumplings one evening. I shook my head. He didn't need to always hear the truth, but he would never hear a lie from me.

All of Samantha's clothes, the short little dresses, the nine-inch heels, were stuffed in a green recyclable bag from Coles under my bed. Every time I walked into my bedroom, I would see a heel poking out from under the bed, or a twinkle of gold from a sparkly dress. I'd get a flashback of a dark boudoir, a man lying on the bed in a white towel, me undressing seductively . . . yes, those memories made me smile, that life seemed so long ago! But it also made me feel uncomfortable. I am not sure why. A constant reminder of Samantha's demise was teasing me daily. Did she fail? Could she have handled her role better? Why did the show have to end so badly?

But like any relationship demise, I didn't want the memories hanging around, so I threw the bag in the back of my car and the next time I drove past Vinnies, I dumped it at the door, along with broken TV sets and plastic bags of kids' clothes. It was hard not to giggle at the thought of some earnest volunteer cautiously pulling out my clothes and shoes, one by one, the odd sexy bra and crotchless set, and wondering what story they told.

'What are you going to do now?' Tab asked during an idle afternoon with our coffees. 'I mean, you've got to start earning money soon. What about going back to magazines? You were so good at it. Yeah, go on! Go back to beauty! I could do with some new products.'

We had a laugh, but she was right. Money was running out and while, sure, I could do with more skincare samples, it was bit more serious than that. The thought of commuting into the city again, fighting the traffic, dropping the kids off stressed, picking them up late and still stressed, for a few hundred bucks a day, before tax, no longer interested me. I know most mums work, and I respect that, but now I had the taste of the money and the freedom – could I really take a step back? The glamour and façade of the magazine world had more than lost its shine.

Magazines were either closing or blending, meaning job cuts. Wages, which hardly paid the bills at the best of times, were being frozen and people were nervous about their future in the industry. Why on earth would I want to go back to that?

I could set up my own business (in what though?), I could claim Centrelink (not a chance). I could get a rich boyfriend (done that – nothing's free).

Or Samantha could come out to play.

No she couldn't.

Yes she could.

No! I threw her clothes away! She's gone!

You can always buy more. You never liked that cheap crap anyway.

She was assaulted. She's broken. She's over it!

Actually, no. She didn't lose her empowerment; she became stronger. She didn't die that afternoon in room 6. She was reborn.

Samantha was ready to come back. Not in the same way – reincarnation doesn't create the same person again and again. Her character has changed and evolved, taking in every droplet of knowledge she learnt along the way, ready for the next journey.

Once I had justified it to myself, and I'd done the annoying dance of should I, shouldn't I, I knew I was ready.

Samantha was coming back. I just wasn't sure how.

The Middle Eastern dinners and sport on TV was only ever going to be a passing fad. Not that I didn't like the boy with the dog. He was awesome. I was just getting itchy, twitchy. Comfortable coupledom didn't suit me any better now than it did before. It wasn't the right time for love. 'I'm sorry,' I explained, and he understood. After three months of wearing thongs and denim shorts, of sitting in cafés or on the beach, it was time to head back to the office – the kind of office I was used to.

Here I was again, scouring the back pages, looking for something to spark my interest. I saw ads for massage places, and I hear it paid well, but I had tiny wrists. I was never going to be any good.

Another Bordello-type place? Look, once you've worked in the best, it's hard to go down a notch. I didn't end up calling any.

A high-class agency? Hmm.

'How old are you?' the lady behind the desk said, staring at me. She was beautiful, Russian and blonde. This was an agency for the elite – or so it said. It certainly was busy. I could hear phones going constantly from another room, a stressed-out receptionist trying to accommodate the needs of lonely men.

'Thirty-five,' I replied, staring back at her, knocking four years off my true age. I was old hat now; I even knew how to lie!

'Hmm, ve vill say 30,' she replied, marking it off on a piece of paper.

'How tall are you?' was the next question.

'Five foot seven,' I replied.

'Hmm. Ve vill say five nine.' Another scribble on her paper.

'Vat colour is your hair?' she asked, now staring at my hair.

Um, was this a trick question? Couldn't she see the colour of my hair?

'Er, brunette? I mean sunkissed?' I stammered. Should I have said blonde?

'Ve vill change ze colour of your hair, you vill be happy with that?' she asked.

'Er, yes of course,' I replied, but my heart felt heavy. Peroxide never suited me.

'Vat you vant from this job?' she asked.

'I want to work hard and makes lots of money.'

'Okay. Ve vill vant you 24/7. You vill make lots of money here. You vill travel the world. Ve have girls here lining up the day they turn 18 begging us to give zem a job. You vill be happy and ve vill be happy. But ve vill vant you to sleep with your phone by your bed. Do you understand?'

'Yes that is fine, but I can only work one week on, and one week off. I have children.'

'Ah. That may be problem for us. Maybe, maybe not. I vant you to meet ze owner. He vill like you. Come back tomorrow and I make sure he is there.'

But I didn't go back. As tempting as it sounded, I couldn't let someone else run my life. I didn't want to have to sleep with my phone, or change the colour of my hair based on someone else's preference.

It was time to go it alone.

I could be a private girl. I'd seen and acted in one part of the sex industry, now it was time to experience another. I was pretty high class before, but now, I was going elite. A good journalist needs to investigate all sides of the story before she can write a well-balanced and well-researched story. That's what I told myself anyway – if only I believed it.

Samantha was upgrading.

I rented a unit in a nice part of town, and I invested in some expensive designer clothes. I advertised on a website well-known by gentlemen who preferred class and companionship over quick walk-in appointments.

My price was high. I wasn't the most expensive girl on the website, but I definitely wasn't the cheapest. I charged what I felt I was worth, what I knew I was worth. And it was considerably more than what I had been getting at The Bordello.

My costs were high enough to justify it.

Forget the daily costs of kids, food and bills. My job cost me money.

Hair: $1200 every three months

Face: Botox and fillers, $1500 every six months

Brows and lashes: approx. $200 every month

Not to mention clothes, shoes, manis, pedis, the waxing. It was exhausting and expensive creating an extremely high-end Samantha. I wouldn't be taking my Louboutins to Vinnies. Ever.

I used the same photos that The Bordello had used and I called myself the same name. (It was more a chance to annoy them than anything else.) I purchased a second phone, got a second phone number and a different email address. And Samantha was ready to rock and roll.

SAMANTHA
A promotion

One of the reasons most working girls don't go into private work is because of the ridiculous amount of admin involved.

'Babe, do it. You'll be great,' breathed a very sexy Asian one evening, before I left The Bordello. We were discussing other avenues within the sex industry. 'I did it and charged $800 an hour, but I had to leave because I couldn't cope with the admin.'

'The ad men?' Was she just attracting men from advertising agencies?

'Yeah, babe, the admin. The constant phone calls, texts and messages all times of the day. The time-wasters. Babe, there were so many time-wasters. I might make less money here but at least I don't have to deal with the men.'

I didn't really believe her. How hard could it be? Dealing with a few texts and emails. It was hardly rocket science.

I didn't get what she meant until I experienced it. She was spot on.

One man from Melbourne went to the trouble of emailing me three times to try to tie up his business trip with me. We worked out a date. He sent me messages leading up to the date like *Can't wait to see you* and *6 more sleeps*, then *2 more sleeps!*

He told me which hotel he would be staying at, told me what time to be there, and that he had booked a nice seafood place for dinner. He even asked me what wine I would like. And then, on the actual day of his highly anticipated date, he went AWOL.

He didn't respond to my voicemail messages. He ignored my texts. He seemed to have disappeared off the face of the earth, leaving me with my face made up, my hair perfect, wearing a nice new outfit and very confused. 'Sorry,' I mumbled to my nanny. 'The date's cancelled.'

A few weeks later, I couldn't resist it. I emailed him. 'Hey Nick, I'm curious to know what happened to you that night? Did you die or did you just bottle it?'

No response from that one either. Who knows what happened to him – did he get a better offer? Or was the fun in the chase, the arranging? Or maybe he did die.

Not that I had much time to think about it. Business was booming! I was inundated with requests, bookings and meetings. Some cancelled, most didn't.

Samantha was a bit different now. I had gone elite and I was beginning to act like it. Clients weren't clients in my language any more; they were 'gentlemen'.

I had a strict no-drugs policy; my unit was even non-smoking. I didn't want any troubled souls lighting up crystal meth. It makes me shudder now to think back to what I saw at The Bordello. No, my clients were all class. Instead of cheap spirits and dirty mirrors, we enjoyed a glass or two of fine wine, or a good scotch. Mostly they requested water – sparkling of course – with a dash of lemon and some ice. *Clink clink.* Cheers, darling! Here's to us.

The men I was meeting now were the big boys of the city. Bankers, accountants, but they didn't just work in an office. They owned it. Their time was precious. They didn't want to waste it parking their Audis and Porsches, walking through a reception area and sitting in some waiting room, having already been seen by a dozen or so eyes. They were short on time yet big on discretion. These men wouldn't go to The Bordello. Half of them hadn't even heard of it.

I didn't think I could love a job more than The Bordello. But I was beginning to wonder why the hell I didn't really think of this private work before. I was my own boss (but this time, *really* my own boss); I was meeting a higher standard of men (none of my clients smoked, let alone did drugs) and I really did only work when I wanted to. I didn't have to sit through annoyingly addictive daytime TV anymore, no more being on tenterhooks as to whether I was going to get fired. No more heated microwave meals. I could take myself off to the gourmet food hall at David Jones! And I was seeing far fewer men, maybe one or two a day if that, and making more money. This was better. This was more me.

It felt quite weird getting ready in the mornings, putting on a suit and 'going to work' and heading to the city (on my time). No messy open-plan office, but a little place of my own: a queen-sized bed and selection of fine drinks, with an indoor pool on level 1 and a gym, nestled between cafés and restaurants.

At lunch-time, I'd take myself off for a stroll to the shops, brushing the side of anxious office workers busily walking past, out of breath, smoking, in a rush, on their phones, while I ambled past, looking into shop windows, smiling to myself that I only had one more client today, and that wasn't for another hour, so why not treat myself to a nice glass of Moët and some oysters. And oh, look! A sale! Those shoes look rather nice . . .

The clients had some bizarre requests. 'So this is where they hide out, in the private world,' I smiled to myself, responding to yet another request for a golden shower (denied). The oddest perhaps was from a man who wanted me to wear a sanitary pad. He loved the feel and texture of them, apparently. And of course, men being the visual creatures they are, he also sent me a photo of himself wearing one (unrequested, I hasten to add), because that is just the sort of photo I like to receive while enjoying my first morning coffee of the day in my gym gear with my dogs at my feet. 'I wear one every day to work,' he wrote – almost proudly.

'Really?' I wrote back, half-amused. 'What do you do for work?'

'I'm in construction.'

Jesus, really? I squinted, pulled the phone closer to have a look. True to his word, I could make out a flick of neon from his jacket, the rolled-down navy trousers and the top of his dusty boots. And of course, I could most definitely see the panty pad protruding out of his boxer shorts.

It was hard not to be shocked – or at least laugh. A big tough tradie wearing a panty pad under his neons was the last thing *anyone* would expect, even me.

Needless to say, we didn't meet up.

I had my period.

*

If I learnt about marriage in The Bordello, I learnt about wealth as a private girl. It didn't matter how rich a man was, or what top elitist school his kids attended, or whether he had just come back from taking the family to Aspen, these men were still unsatisfied with their lives and relationships. In my eye there was no difference between the man who baulked at the prices The Bordello offered or the men who would hand me four of five times the amount. Most were lonely and most were looking for something more than a quick fuck, although one client did confess his wife hadn't touched his penis for 20 years. They were looking for longer-term companion-ship, for a girlfriend who was 'theirs' but who didn't put any demands on them. I swear some saw it as a dating service for pretty girls and wealthy men – and in a way, it was. I was quite glad of that; I was happy to be someone's concubine.

Bankers were the oddest breed. Most were nice; a few, well, I'd call them quirky. I put it down to the stress of their job. One lovely man in his thirties, six-foot-three with tanned skin, visited me for just a massage, no sex and no kissing (he had a fiancée at home). He told me that half the banking world were snorting cocaine up their noses to get through the long days and nights. 'I don't really want to do drugs but a colleague offered me some one evening and I tried it. I didn't realise how many of my friends were on the stuff day-in, day-out. They need it to just get through.' Call me naive but I had no idea. What kind of pressure were these poor people under? No wonder they needed a form of release.

It made sense, though, when I soon got to experience their behaviour. One high-flyer emailed me his photo straight after our first contact, and told me he had a spare few hours as he was waiting for the Hong Kong markets to open. He gave me his full name, where he lived, and told me he was married with two older kids, was looking for a long-term companion and was I open to that? Bear in mind, I had never met this man, we had never conversed. He had just seen my profile and photos (face non-identifiable) and had taken it I was 'the one' for him.

Before I even had time to reply, he had sent me another photo: a smiling, reasonably good-looking man wearing a Polo shirt and a Tag watch, his arm draped casually over a chair, clearly at a sports match of some kind, with his gold wedding ring staring at me.

'Hey, this is me!' he wrote. 'What do you think? Reckon you would like to be my only girl? I want to look after you – you seemed perfect for me. God, this is crazy – I haven't even met you but I feel you're the right girl. I'm so tempted to give you an apartment in the city plus keys to my new sports Merc.'

And so it went on. I wasn't sure how to play it. I didn't want his unit in the city or his car. It was odd that he was throwing his identity and his possessions at someone he hadn't even met, or spoken to.

I played along with it, intrigued as ever, and we arranged to meet. He was taking me to dinner at one of the finest restaurants in Sydney. But there was one request from this gentleman. Would I mind awfully if he brought an outfit for me to wear?

This was new. 'Sure,' I typed back, enjoying this game. 'But show me a photo please.'

I'm not sure what I was expecting – maybe something short but classy. Tight but demure. When the photo came through, I almost let out a scream.

A red rubber catsuit. Was he fucking serious?

This client wanted me to wear a red PVC catsuit to one of Sydney's premier dining establishments. The place he was taking me to wasn't young and funky, it was iconic. You wouldn't find reality pop stars there, you'd be dining with prime ministers and premiers. If I turned up in a red rubber catsuit, I'd either be shown the door pretty quickly, or they would have had me arrested. By the fashion police.

Shit, how was I going to handle this one? This client might be great, but the catsuit? Rubber? Red? Imagine if I bumped into a parent from the school? 'Whoops sorry, I thought this was a Halloween party.' An unlikely excuse, considering it was April.

'What do you think? Sexy, huh?' he wrote. The hope in his words practically leapt out at me. 'I would love it if you would wear this for our meal together!'

What could I say? I didn't want to hurt his feelings. But I was surprised that a man who lived and worked in a corporate world would choose such an outfit for dinner.

He was married – wasn't he worried about being seen? We would hardly fade into the background or go unnoticed. I would be the bloody laughing stock of Sydney's elite diners.

'Do you have anything else slightly less conspicious?' I typed cautiously. 'As stunning and sexy is this is, I just would feel a bit uncomfortable in this outfit at such-and-such restaurant.' Ahem.

Then came the next photo. This time, a black PVC dress, so tight it would have shown my varicose veins. It wasn't hard to work out his fetish. But at least it was black. I could wear stockings. I could wear a long coat.

'Okay,' I replied. 'Drop it at the reception of the hotel and I will pick it up.'

'Wonderful, thank you,' he wrote. 'See you Thursday at 7.'

Thursday at 7 arrived. The client hadn't responded to my messages since morning. Was he wrapped in rubber somewhere with an orange in his mouth? Had his wife found out and attacked him with the Gladwrap?

Another one who had vanished. What a strange lot they were! To be honest, I couldn't help but feel relieved. Though the bastard could have let me know – I'd been fasting since midday to have the flattest stomach possible for that bloody rubber.

It was beginning to be a bit of a habit now. Something men did, this wasting of my time. Maybe they were trying to see whether I'd accept the challenge. Maybe it was just a game to them.

Or maybe their behaviour was the result of too much cocaine, too much money and too much stress. The rubber man was not alone in his time-wasting manner – there were many more like him. It was hard not to take it personally – was it me? Did they change their minds because of something I did wrong? Maybe the whole banking fraternity was sitting around together, scheming on how to get private girls excited then dump them at the 11th hour. (I can assure you boys, there is nothing exciting about a red spray-on rubber catsuit to a woman the wrong side of 35.)

But for every weird one, there was also a perfect gentleman. Men who came into your life for a reason, men whom you felt were made for you. And in this game, dear friends, that only means one thing. Feelings. And that is never, ever a good thing.

There is a private job I do that involves crabsticks. Relax. Melvin and the Ferrero Rocher was a lesson learnt and Samantha has never said yes to food in her appointments again. I don't even do chocolate-flavoured condoms.

Do you know I can't even look at those chocolates now? But they seem to pop up in my life all the time, ever since Melvin.

It's a bit like when a boyfriend called James, for example, dumps you and now everything you see is James-related. James Street, James Removals, James and Co Real Estate.

I was in my newsagent's, having a perfectly pleasant conversation about something or other with the man who works behind the counter, when he turned round and made a rustling sound from a plastic bag.

'Here, darling,' he said in broken English, passing me something small. 'A leetle present for you.' He gently pressed something in my hand, a little brown chocolate, wrapped in gold and brown paper.

'Oh – thank you,' I replied, blinking at the hard little Ferrero Rocher in my hand, hoping the disgust wasn't written on my face.

'Aren't you lucky?' smiled the old lady behind me. 'Who doesn't love Ferrero Rocher!'

I chucked it in the bin instead.

Another time, in the local supermarket at Christmas time, everyone was in a joyous mood, stocking up on ham and chutney. 'Amanda!' cried the manager, a friend of mine. 'Something for you! Happy Christmas, darling!' And handed me a plastic clear box of little chocolates, yep, you've guessed it.

'Oh thanks, Andrew,' I replied, faking a smile. 'My *favourite.*'

'Yeah, all the girls love a bit of Ferrero Rocher,' he winked back.

I shot him a look – but nah. How could he know?

I gave them to my cleaners.

You're waiting for the crabstick story, aren't you? Don't worry, you can carry on eating. As if I would allow a crabstick to go anywhere near me now! Dahling, didn't you know? I'm high class now! Oysters all the way!

There are these three accountants. Three lovely, lovely men. All married, all in their fifties, and all living nice, little neat lives with large rambling houses in the south, with big outdoor pools and fancy cars.

I wouldn't say they were Dom Pérignon, but sparkling Prosecco.

We meet every three months in a serviced apartment in the city – whichever has the best deal at the time. These meetings are always pre-arranged and given lots of thought and planning. It's not just me who meets them, there are three gentlemen, and three girls, in a three-bedroom unit and I have been part of this secret ring for over a year now.

When I was first asked to attend, by a girl called Nessie whom I'd worked with at Lola's, I was petrified. I thought it was going to be all gang bangs, swapping, viewing, lesbian sex and so forth. That wasn't my style.

'You'll be fine,' reassured Nessie. 'They're harmless, lovely guys. It's mostly about the lunch. Will you do it?'

My ears pricked up. Lunch? Now you're talking. I knew the code. This was going to be an appointment at an exclusive restaurant, with a seafood platter and champagne on ice. We'd get a bit tipsy on the finest before tip-toeing into a five-star hotel each with a handsome businessman linked in our arms. This was what it was all about. I'd seen Billie Piper on *The Secret Diary of a London Call Girl* and that was her life, wasn't it? Now it was mine.

I deserved to be wined and dined. Obviously Nessie had clocked onto the type of classy girl I was; I knew there was a reason I always liked her. She could see I was different; sophisticated. A cut about the rest.

'All right,' I replied, 'just give me the address and I will be there on the day. What shall I wear?'

'Oh casual is fine. They're just normal guys. Jeans and a nice top.'

Ha. I could read between lines. These men were very important. They were probably recognised wherever they went due to the high-profile roles they had in the business word. They needed discretion, class and maturity. Something classic, designer . . . I'm thinking David Jones for this one, not Myer.

The details were revealed over the next few days. We'd be at a serviced apartment near Chinatown.

This was looking up. They'd probably booked some table at Quay. Or Cafe Sydney. A short taxi ride anyway – easy.

'Yes, I think I know.'

'Yeah, meet me there, at reception. Bill will come and get us and show us to the room.'

'And then we have lunch?'

'Oh yes, don't worry – the lunch is the main part of the day. It's always more about the eating and company than it is the sex – you know that already Sammy. We'll have a nice lunch, and lots of wine, so don't drive!'

Oh yummy! I hadn't been to a nice restaurant for a while. This was the sort of place you went with someone you loved, or at least liked a lot. And I hadn't felt that in ages.

I primped and pampered, I even had a spray tan. The glare of some of these restaurants can be so harsh on one's skin!

I didn't eat much the morning of The Lunch. Avocado on toast, just one piece. 'Not hungry today, Amanda?' my local barista commented, raising an eyebrow at my uneaten breakfast.

'I'm having a big lunch,' I grinned back, patting my tummy.

At 1 pm it was time to go. I hopped in a taxi, and off I went. Should I have the bread roll? I thought, checking my lipstick as we sped past all the regular people eating their lunch in pokey cafés. Probably not. I've farted in a booking before and could have sworn it was the wheat. Mind you, the nice bread rolls at those places on the water are usually the home-made, melt-in-your-mouth kind . . .

'Hey Sammy,' smiled Ness, kissing my cheek when I found her. 'You look lovely. Bill said we can go straight up.'

'Great!' I smiled. 'I'm starving, aren't you?'

'Sure am,' she winked, as we waited for the lift.

I couldn't see it at first when I walked into the apartment. A sea of heads popped in front of me to say hello. Kiss, kiss, kiss.

'I'm Bill!'

'I'm Ben!'

'And I'm Brent! Welcome to our gang, Samantha!'

They weren't the most handsome lot in the world – one was wearing a zip-up bum bag around his waist – but they were treating us to lunch and seemed awfully sweet. Wasn't this lovely? Wasn't I lucky?

'Hello gentlemen,' I replied, pecking each one on the lips. 'I just wanted to say thank you for lunch – what a lovely idea. I've been practically starving myself all week!'

Bill squeezed my bottom. 'Oh that's good,' he said, showing me to the table. 'Because we've got plenty here. Come on, throw your jacket off, darlin'. Tuck in! The chicken's straight from Coles; it'll get cold if you don't have some now. Ben, can you chuck me the packet of prawns? And that jar of herrings? Didn't we buy Burger Rings too, or just those Twisties?'

I must have looked like Paris Hilton just dropped off on a muddy farm. My mouth must have dropped open and I must have looked completely gutted.

'What's the matter, love? You're not one of those veggos are ya? Jesus, Brent, we've got a carrot muncher on our hands here; a little bunny rabbit! Don't worry, love, I think we picked up one of those deli salads too, a creamy pasta one with greens in it. We never let anyone go home hungry here. I'll open the lid for you. The nice lady at the deli even gave us some cutlery. Now where is it?'

There were crabsticks, Coles-brand hummus, some olives and a nice stick of fluorescent white French bread that snapped like a brittle bone as I took a piece.

Samantha might be a food snob, but she was never, ever rude. 'Mmm,' I mumbled, trying to chew my food. 'This is delicious.'

The afternoon wasn't that bad, more like a scene from my parents' favourite comedy shows. If only they could see how hilarious this job was sometimes. If only people knew what really went on in this world. Sex swinging from chandeliers? I wish. Where the hell were the clients Billie Piper had? The cosmetic surgeons, the hot cops? I got three balding accountants with a taste for herring rollmops.

The accountants were very sweet men, and their priority was not only the sex (which consisted usually of no more than fifteen minutes in our six-hour bookings), but also conversations, wine and always lots of, um, food.

And the routine was always the same. Bang on 4 pm, it was tea time. 'Better get the kettle on,' Bill would say, pulling himself out of bed. 'I think Brent's got some dessert from memory, cheesecake was on special this week . . . how do you like your tea, love?'

'Strong,' I replied. 'Very, very strong.'

The last hour was always spent stacking the dishwasher, draining the bottles of wine and arguing about who should – or in my case shouldn't – take the scraps of some poor battery-hen chicken home.

'Go on darling, you take it, there's enough there for a salad,' Bill would say earnestly, wrapping the stinking carcass in a plastic bag, pushing it in my direction, far too close for comfort.

'No, Bill, really, I won't eat it, let's just put it in the bin,' I would always reply, with a slight edge to my voice.

But they were genuine blokes, and salt of the earth. They adored their wives and just needed fun in the way of pretty girls and 'lunch', every few months.

On one occasion, a week or so before Christmas, we had another one of our lunches booked. By now I'd had five or so of these culinary feasts under my belt, and I knew what to expect. So more often than not, I'd eat before I went, and just nibble at the salads. Sometimes I would bring in my own food. The chicken always made me feel a bit sick – the stench of the meat, the heat coming from the plastic bag. How many hands had touched this food? It made my stomach turn.

This time, I raised an eyebrow when I saw the table. It had been laid out already, with Yuletide crackers and silly party hats. That wasn't even the most shocking part. There was a neat plate of something green and tasty-looking, admittedly still suffocating in Gladwrap, carefully tucked behind the crabsticks and herring rollmops.

'Ohh! Dolmades, Bill?' I exclaimed teasingly, smiling. That was a bit posh, wasn't it? They were certainly pushing the boat out for this merry occasion.

'I know, love,' he replied excitedly, pecking me on the cheek. 'But it is Christmas after all.'

Chapter Fifteen

AMANDA
Never too old

I seem to attract conversations about sex wherever I go. Just now, waiting at Gold Coast airport to head back to Sydney, I start up a conversation with a New Zealander sitting next to me.

'What book are you reading?' I ask her, peering over her shoulder.

'Ah, some crap,' she smiled, showing me the cover. 'I don't care, I love reading. I always need to have a book with me. Except that *Fifty Shades of Grey* book – oh no, that wasn't for me. I was too embarrassed to buy it.' She started laughing now, shaking her head. 'Imagine the people at the old people's home I work seeing me with that! Mind you, I'm sure half of them would want a copy of it. If only they could read . . .'

We talk for a bit. This lady is a nurse in aged care and spends her eight-hour shift wiping bums and feeding oldies. Now that's a real job. We really didn't have that much in common; what do we talk about? We talk about sex.

'I've got a six-year-old, ten-year-old, 12-year-old and a 20-year-old,' she said, showing me photos. 'My husband wants another, but no way, I'm done.'

'Well at least you're having sex, unlike most married couples,' I replied, nudging her arm.

'Oh sex, don't talk to me about sex. The old ducks in the home go crazy for sex.'

My ears pricked up. Now, this was interesting. 'Oh? Do tell.'

'We have a 90-year-old who can't stop playing with her you-know-what. She keeps rubbing it on the edge of her chair. I told the other nurses we need to order in some dildos. I need to get her one before she explodes. We have a married couple in their nineties who are still at it. We constantly hear their bed rocking in the night. And then there's Percy; lovely Percy, 95, and we order in one of those, you know, sex workers every bloody week to give him a good bloody shag. Horny as a rabbit on heat, that one. You'd think they would get over all that by the time they get to their age, wouldn't you?'

I was crying with laughter now. Why is my life always surrounded by stories like this?

'That is hilarious,' I told her. 'Seriously funny, thank you.' Our flight was being called and we queued up together.

'And don't get me started on full moons,' she went on, draining the last of her flat white. 'They are all horny as hell when there's a full moon. We have to keep a good watch on them in case the place turns into a bloody orgy. When I work nights, I often have to lock the doors of the bedrooms as some of the old blokes go wandering round the ward for sex. Half those women would say yes but there would be too much mess for us to clear up.'

God this was funny. And I can believe it, too. Did this game of cat and mouse ever end? According to this Florence Nightingale, sex is a part of us, a big part of us, until we die.

We parted ways as we went to find our separate seats.

As I clicked on my seatbelt and settled in, I was still smiling. Sex workers at old people's homes . . . horny pensioners . . . and then the thought suddenly hit me. Should I have given her my business card?

SAMANTHA
Saggy bums

There's always at least one horrible experience. One man who ruins it. At The Bordello there was the assault, and in the world of privates, there was Alan.

Alan told me he was 37. He worked in finance (of course) and was divorced (not hard to work out why when I got to know him). He booked an appointment to see me at noon on a weekday for an hour.

The same day I happened to be in the world's slowest taxi. We seemed to slow down at the green lights and pootle along in the slow lane as if we were going on a Sunday drive with a nice picnic hamper in the boot.

I tried to catch the driver's attention, but it was a bit hard to distract him from the influx of calls he was taking on his mobile, speaking in a hushed mumble in some foreign language.

How far away R U Samantha? beeped the text from Alan.

Christ, he was early. And it looked like I was going to be late. That was it. The driver's scintillating conversation with his mother would have to be interrupted.

'Look, sorry if this sounds rude but I have a very important meeting at 12. Do you mind if you drive a bit faster?' I hated sounding like this but if there was one thing I was learning about men in the CBD, it was that they had no time to waste.

'Yes, yes, sorry,' laughed the driver, hanging up. But we still crept along the quiet roads, with geriatrics in Holden Barinas speeding past us.

Sorry, Alan, I may be five minutes late, I texted, glancing at my watch. It was 11.40. I would probably make it but just wanted to give Alan some notice just in case.

Really? came the reply. *I am disappointed, Samantha, that you will be five minutes late to an appointment I made six hours ago.*

Shit. He was playing hardball. But fair call. He was right; there was no excuse for me leaving at the last minute. I was dealing with the big boys now. I had to lift my game.

'So what do you do for work?' asked the driver, trying not to look at my cleavage, and giving me a flash of his nicotine-stained teeth.

For fuck's sake just DRIVE! I wanted to scream. But instead, I smiled sweetly. 'I'm a writer,' I seethed through gritted teeth. For Christ's sake, put your foot down! There are no cars in front of us, go go GO! Shit, what a surprise. Another red light.

The driver turned round to me and grinned. 'Ohh! A writer! What are you writing, Miss?'

I smiled the most sarcastic smile I could manage, but I never liked to be rude. 'Nothing at the moment,' I snapped.

What's your ETA Samantha? came another text. Heart pumping, stomach turning. I didn't want to lose this client. I had barely started my business – I didn't want to come across as unprofessional.

We weren't going to make it, I was sure of that. *I'm awfully sorry Alan, I would hate to stuff you around. It's best we reschedule. Alan for your inconvenience, I would like to offer you a 50% discount if you decide to book again with me. I am terribly sorry,* I wrote. This bloody taxi driver had cost me a job.

Thanks, I appreciate that, he wrote back and that I thought was that.

But Alan clearly had nothing else to do that day. He kept on messaging, showing off that he was being sent to Hong Kong for work for a week 'but they will probably extend'. Yeah, yeah, you're so smart, I thought.

But I felt I had to go along with it, because of my guilt at stuffing him around. *Oh you're so clever!* I wrote back, or something to that effect. *And sexy too!*

Are you filthy? Do you want me to fuck you hard?'

Oh yes, darling, I wrote back, while sitting on the loo, reading *New Idea*. 'I'd love that . . .'

And on it went. All day. By 5 that evening I was tired and he was boring me.

Do U need more cock tonight? came the text when I was on my way home. Oh for God's sake, didn't he have anything else in his life? What did he do before I came along? Cock was the last thing on my mind, especially his pencil dick. I wanted a cup of tea, a few squares of chocolate and a cuddle with my dogs.

No darling, I'm going to bed, goodnight.

You don't want to come to my house and let me fuck you hard?

240

He was annoying me now, going from client I needed to appease to revolting pest. He clearly had nothing better to do than text someone he had never met. I was tired, mentally drained and over it.

Do you work all night for free? I wrote, moodily now. In other words: Fuck off mate.

What do you mean? Of course I had to explain to this imbecile.

It means I am not working now, I'm going home goodnight.

It wouldn't be for free, it would be for money.

Yes I realise that. Anyway, I feel bad about our appointment and I promise I will make it up to you. Enjoy your trip.

Make it up to me now. You're a naughty girl and need fucking.

And so it went on. He had said he was 37. Did he mean 17?

I ended up switching my phone off, only to be woken up in the morning with a *beep beep*.

How are you this morning? Rested and ready to be filthy again?

I rolled my eyes. Jesus, this loser again? *Yes but I am booked out today.*

And then the messages got nasty. Here is an edited version of the conversation that ensued in the next few hours.

One of my friends booked you and the feedback was not that great. You look 40 plus . . . you have stretch marks on your stomach most likely from kids . . . you've got a saggy ass . . . you've got a bogan tattoo . . . a droopy fanny . . .

I typed my response. *I hope you feel better in yourself for saying this Alan.*

Another old dog who thinks she is 20. Get real and look in the mirror. Try going to the gym!!! My mate said you were horrible!!!! No guys want an old single mum with stretch marks ... I'm going to write a bad review of you when I am in Hong Kong, he wrote back.

Please don't contact me again Alan.

Ouch, ouch, triple ouch. Did I really look over the hill? I checked my reflection in the mirror; was my bum a bit saggy? As for my 'droopy fanny' – what the hell did that mean? It was laughable, if only I wasn't so sensitive.

Maybe he was right, I was a fraud. Who was I kidding? Is that how these men saw me? As a saggy old wrinkly stretch-marked single mother? Part of me was indignant that someone who had never met me could be so horrible. I could never speak to someone like that.

But there was a bigger part of me that hung onto every word he said and believed it. He was right; I was old. I said in my profile I was 34, not about to turn 40.

'Jesus Christ!' Tab said when I called her in tears. With her counselling background, she's always good in an emotional crisis. Never one to coddle, I could always rely on my darling Tab to be straight-up.

'Amanda! You know that's not true. You've got to toughen up. You've got bookings coming out of your ears and most of your clients are repeat customers. Why are you listening to this dickhead who has never even met you? Get over it!'

Pause.

'And what did he say about your fanny again?'

Sniff. 'It was droopy.' Sniff.

'That's bloody funny, Amanda. Come on, droopy fanny? Cheer up!'

You're probably laughing too. But if you were a nurse, imagine someone telling you the way you handled that patient was appalling. Imagine if you were a teacher and the parents of your students started talking about how you were the worst teacher ever. My body was my business. Tab could have said anything, but her words fell on deaf (wrinkly, saggy, stretch-marked) ears. I went to a clattery café in the city to calm down, but tears dropped into my latte as I re-read his black-and-white words on my phone.

Why was I getting so upset about this? Alan and I had never met. I had upset him by making it crystal clear that he was a pest, but I didn't deserve this abuse. It was hurtful. It annoyed me that I was so upset. But his words were mean and spiteful, and I wasn't used to hearing such nastiness.

I couldn't work today. Me and my decrepit body were going home. I didn't have the energy to shout for a taxi. I just waved my pathetic little arms in the air and flagged one. Here's goes another annoying ride.

'Bondi Junction, please,' I said sadly to the taxi driver – this time a female. Thank God. I was in no mood for nicotine teeth this afternoon.

She nodded and I sat in the back, masking my tears.

Another old dog who think she's 20.

Actually, I never pretend to be 20. My clients come to me because I'm mature.

Get to the gym.

I go to the gym!

You've got stretch marks all over your tummy, you've got a saggy ass . . .

Enough! Did he think I don't have those voices in my head already? Don't most of us? Our legs, our bums, our tums, the way we do our job, the way we parent, the way we do everything. Don't we all try and counteract the little negative voice that sits on our shoulder all day whispering 'You're not good enough'?

Who hasn't thought at least once in their life that they're a fraud and any second now, someone is going to find out and expose them? I know I certainly have those thoughts. And Alan, that nasty piece of work whoever he is, had just confirmed all my little nasty fears. Just because he didn't get what he wanted, when he wanted it.

How could I get naked with a new client now? How could I gain the confidence to meet a new man?

I was just building my business up. The self-doubt came up in waves. Maybe I was deluded to think I could do this.

Then the tears started to roll. I couldn't help it. It's not often Samantha, or Amanda, feels much, but I felt something now. Hurt, self-loathing or a desperate panic as to how the fuck I had ended up in this taxi, in this situation, in the first place. I shed tears about my parents, about my life. I'd fucked everything up. I was a mess. My life was a mess. I'd had everything: a husband, the house, the part-time job in magazines. I was a great journalist and a great writer. And I gave it all up to be a bloody hooker. What the fuck was I thinking? Jesus Christ. I wound the window down, gasping for fresh air. Was this reality slapping me in my wrinkly old face?

'What's up with you love?' snapped the taxi driver, furrowing her brows at me in the mirror.

'Nothing,' I whispered, wiping my tears.

'What it is? Man trouble?'

I shook my head, trying to find my voice, which now sounded more like a croak. 'I'm an escort . . . horrible man . . . sent me messages . . . saggy arse . . .' I pointed to my phone and burst into tears again, disrupted only by the shudder of the car as my driver slammed on the brakes. We had, it seemed, pulled up on the side of the road just outside Bondi Junction. I went to get out, but with a click the doors locked.

'Now listen here, love,' she said, turning round to face me. 'I'm 56 years old. I've been driving cabs for 20 years. You don't think I've heard enough shit like this from men? You don't think I get this shit on a day-to-day basis?'

Shocked, I nodded. Where was this going? I took my sunglasses off to meet her eyes.

'Now, you think I let it get to me? You think I sit down and cry every time I get something nasty thrown at me? Listen 'ere, and listen 'ere good. For whatever reason, you've chosen a tough industry. Men are going to judge you on the way you look all the time. You need to toughen up, girl; grow some balls. You can't cry every time a man gives you some shit. If I did that, I'd be a blubbering mess.'

I nodded again, feeling better already. God bless this woman.

'Okay, thank you,' I whispered, leaning forwards to get out.

'No you don't,' she snapped, scaring me. 'You're not getting out of this car until I hear you say something for me. Will you say it, love?'

'Yes?'

'Garbage in, garbage out. Say it. It's an affirmation I say to myself every morning and every night. SAY IT.'

'Garbage in, garbage out,' I whispered shyly, looking down. Jesus, why did I always end up in these situations?

'Come on! I didn't hear you. Say it louder. I want you to look at me and say it three times to me before I let you out.'

I brought my eyes up to hers. Of course I started crying again, this time, not from someone's nastiness but from their kindness. 'Garbage in, garbage out, garbage in, garbage out, garbage in, garbage out.'

'That's me girl,' she chuckled, and clicked the doors open for me. I paid her. 'Thank you,' I said quietly, but this time I smiled at her. To this day, I will never forget Chris the taxi driver, and her kindness. There really are angels in disguise walking amongst us. And they happen to fly into our lives just when we need them.

She was a tough old bird. Driving cabs couldn't be easy. The types of drunk idiots she would have had to pick up in her taxi late on Saturday nights made me shudder. If she could be strong, so could I. Sure, my body isn't microscopically perfect but I never said it was. I like who I am, and I do a good job. I make people happy; I make people laugh. And she was right. I had to toughen up. If this was the worst I'd hear in my life, then I've been a lucky girl.

The next day, I was eating Hokkien noodle soup at the David Jones food hall, when a text message pinged. From Alan.

Off to HK now, what successful people do! Enjoy your stretch marks, saggy arse and bogan tats!

This time, I smiled. I even let out a little laugh. 'Waiter!' I called. 'Glass of Moët please, thank you darling.'

'Madam is celebrating something?' smiled the waiter, pouring my glass.

I grinned back. 'Sure am.' Cheers to you, Alan, my guardian angel, Chris, and my squeezable, playful, gorgeously saggy arse!

The incident with Alan the arsehole had shaken me. It was true: I had lied about my age on my profile. I had written I was 34.

I knew I looked 34, but I wasn't. And because I was so bad at maths, I was quite often paranoid that a client would ask what year I was born and of course, panicking at the figures, I would stumble and my silly little lie would be exposed. And as someone who prides themselves in trying to lead an honest life, lying about my age was a bit hypocritical.

So I decided to come clean. I updated my profile. I wrote that I had just turned 40. If age was of utmost importance to my clients, they deserved to know the truth. I also wanted to take the wind out of Alan's sails. He seemed to be fixated on my age, so I wanted to take his power away. While I couldn't really do much about my 'saggy arse, bogan tattoo and droopy fanny' I could at least be honest about my age.

I also wrote I wouldn't see men who lacked manners, plus any harassment would be dealt with quickly and effectively. 'I prefer quality over quantity, instead of more the merrier,' I wrote. I was getting sick of the dickheads who sent me photos of rubber catsuits and dinner plans and then did a disappearing act. Would they act such a twerp to a woman in her forties? One would hope not.

I did wonder of course whether I would ever be booked again. Surely clients were looking for nubile 20-year-olds? Seemingly not. Not only did my clientele increase, but so did the calibre of men. I was no longer getting the time-wasters, the loser Alans of the world, but mature and very successful men were now coming to me. I was getting requests from abroad too: men wanting to book me when they were in town on business. In fact as I am writing this right now, I have just confirmed a booking from a lovely gentleman in San Francisco who would like to take me out to dinner in a month's time when he will be travelling here for work. Men from Adelaide,

Perth, Brisbane and Melbourne contact me in the hope that I'll 'tour' to go and see them.

The men who were choosing me were doing so because they were sick of young girls. They wanted to have a mature and interesting conversation; they wanted experience and sophistication. I could afford to be more picky. I wasn't desperate for clients; business was good.

In fact I turned down clients who were rude, arrogant or too dirty. One client, a medical student who told me he was 30, tried to book me and wrote in great detail how he wanted me to walk around on all fours and bark like a dog.

When he asked my age (he clearly hadn't read my profile), and I told him, he replied: *Hm 40, I am just wondering whether I like older than myself.*

He then wrote: *I'm picky with faces,* followed by, *I am looking forward to meeting you.*

Oh dear. This one I was going to have to let go. I cancelled our booking – much to his disappointment.

Oh no I didn't mean I wanted to cancel, he wrote back quickly. *You misunderstood me.*

Sorry darling, I didn't make myself clear, I typed back. *You're not cancelling our appointment darling, I am. I don't feel comfortable with a client who is unsure whether my age bothers him. I am not in the business of trying to sell myself to you. I certainly do not need to do that . . . the beauty of getting older, darling, is that quite frankly, you know what you want.* In other words, I do not want to see YOU. As much as walking around my unit barking like a bloody Jack Russell seemed such an attractive idea, the answer is no.

One client had an interesting fantasy. He wanted me to meet him at a café and to ask whether I could sit with him.

I had to then tell him how sexy he was and that I've seen him sitting there every day, and could he come upstairs to my unit and fuck me?

It was basically a very public roleplay. I was petrified! I'd never met this man before. He told me he was going to wear a suit and a blue shirt, but when I was walking towards the café, there were at least three men wearing blue shirts sitting there. The last thing I wanted was to get the wrong bloke. Can you imagine?

He would either think he was being set up, or that I was stark raving mad, or that Christmas had come early.

I found my client, said my piece and, true to my word, he followed me to my unit and we fucked. He left after half an hour and I got $600 cash. The reason for his fantasy? His wife had had an affair and he wanted to feel attractive again.

Then I met J. J was a curious client, one whom I still can't make out.

The text message was pretty nondescript. *Hi would you like to spend the night with me at Shangri-La. J.*

J what a lovely invite but I am actually not well and cancelling my bookings tonight. Sorry X.

Very sad. If you feel better call, I want to see no one else.

I switched off my phone. Just another appointment I couldn't make and I didn't think anything more of it.

I wasn't lying, either. I felt bloody awful and couldn't even lift myself off the bed to catch a taxi home.

Back in the day, Amanda would have panicked about brain tumours. But this Amanda had lost her fear over the past couple of years. Was it age? Growing up? Or was it something more? A journey of self-discovery and realisation that actually, I was okay. I didn't feel the need to date a cop or paramedic anymore. I didn't feel like I needed a man who could 'save' me.

Where were my saviours when I was being raped? If nothing else, that experience taught me that I was pretty much good on my own. I didn't need protection from others – that had to come from me. I was strong enough to deal with my demons. I'd survived every hurdle that had come my way. And I was pretty sure I would fight the next one.

So instead of Googling 'headache' and spending the next few hours waiting for impending death, I had a bath and went home. Sorry Mr J, it wasn't meant to be.

A few weeks later: *R u feeling better? J.*

Yes thank you! How thoughtful to remember!

I'd love to meet u this week. I've been intrigued by your profile and haven't seen anyone. How is your schedule?

We agreed on a date, then he sent this.

I would like to meet someone special. Google me, it's xxxxxx. Dinner date would be lovely – happy to keep it financial. I don't want to meet lots of girls, just one my own age that I can spend time with. Could that suit?

J was a big shot in business, that's all that need to be said. Online, he looked like a tall, strong man who wore a suit well. Big plus. More importantly, he sounded reliable and sane. Even bigger plus.

We exchanged a few more texts. He was funny too, compared me to Kim Kardashian and him to Kanye. I liked him and was looking forward to our date. If anything, it would certainly be entertaining.

That's what I loved about this job, especially the private world. The men I met were extremely smart. They worked hard for their success and they were wealthy in monetary values and knowledge too. I could learn something from them. What nuggets of gold would J impart to me?

Would you like my driver to pick you up Samantha? beeped the text message.

I was chatting to one of the shop assistants in a local grocer when that one came through. I tried to feign interest as she was showing me how fresh the parsley was, but that distracted me. A driver? Jesus, who was I, Julia Roberts?

I what a lovely offer and thank you, I would be delighted to accept your kindness. My address is –

Hang on, I thought. Should I be giving a client my address?

This was a client who was worth over $120 million with his own driver and a three-bedroom suite in one of Sydney's most prestigious hotels. What was I going to say, 'Pick me up outside Nando's'?

I told him I'd meet him on the corner of two streets. But I didn't get my hopes up. I'd been through these sorts of things before; I was almost desensitised to it. The driver probably wouldn't show, or the client would text to cancel. Or he just won't respond to my messages and that will be it. Nothing would surprise me.

But bang on 7 pm, a black BMW 7 series glided to our meeting point. My driver, Lin – dressed in a navy suit – was standing in front of my door and when I stepped outside, he smiled and open the door for me.

'Good evening, Samantha,' he said.

It was, seriously, just like *Pretty Woman*. Except I had chosen to wear something a bit more elegant than thigh-high plastic boots.

Oh my fucking *God*. I couldn't hide my smile as I slid into the leather back seat. Were my neighbours watching? I bloody hoped so.

Only 12 hours ago I'd been doing the school run in my Bonds trackies with my hair in a bun, spilling most of my latte on my T-shirt, and now – this. Being swept off my feet by a multimillionaire! And being paid for it! How good was this job!

'Samantha, what time would you like me to take you home?' Lin asked, looking at me through the rearview mirror.

'Midnight,' I replied. 'Thank you, Lin.'

J was handsome and charming and funny. Which wasn't good news for me. I didn't want to *like* him.

But when I knocked on the door of his suite, and this charming man wearing knockabout jeans and a polo shirt answered in bare feet, how could I not think I'd hit the bloody jackpot?

'So here we are!' he smiled, kissing me on the cheek. 'Let me show you around.'

We admired the view, then he showed me the bedroom suite. I noticed all his suits hanging up and smiled at his socks and pants thrown messily on the ground. We kissed on the balcony.

'It's a pretty big place for me by myself,' he whispered in my ear.

'Well, darling, I'm here for the next few hours . . .'

He got up to fix me a drink. 'I have a proposition – if you're open to it, Samantha,' he said, pouring me a glass. I watched as the bubbles fizzed before he handed it over to me.

'I want to give you $10,000 to cancel all your clients this week. Would you be open to that? Is that enough money? Please say if it's not. I just want you to have some time off to think about our future.'

I took a very large sip of champagne and stared at the ceiling. I know I said it takes a lot to shock me these days. But I didn't see this one coming. $10,000?

Our future?

'Okay,' I replied, not wanting to say the wrong thing. 'But what do you want from me in return?' I knew business, and I was beginning to know businessmen.

'I want you to think about us – could we work? I need to buy a house. Would you be open to moving in with me? With your children, of course. I'd want to help raise them.'

I listened incredulously as he discussed it excitedly. He sounded like a teenager planning his first holiday away from his parents. He talked about what he could bring to the table (money, security, love) and what I could bring (I could look after him and the house). 'Your career must come second,' he said.

'Of course,' I replied, playing along with this game, starting to believe it. He wasn't ugly, and he was funny, which was a bonus. And it was impossible to overlook his wealth. I certainly wouldn't need to worry. It was beginning to sound like a jolly good plan to me. Whoops, spilt the champers. I looked in dismay as the wet patch on the carpet grew.

'I'll refill your glass, darling,' he smiled, kissing my nose. 'Plenty more where that came from.'

Oh! I could get used to this. Who couldn't?

We ordered pizza from room service (pancetta and olive), polished off the bottle of Dom and kissed some more, carrying on with the (rich) teenager theme. Then it was time for me to go. Lin was waiting for me.

'Whoops, nearly forgot!' he said. 'Your money.' And he gently took a huge white envelope stuffed with green notes and placed it into my bag. 'Now, darling, give me your word. No clients this week. Use this time to think about our future.'

Cash was beginning to lose its value to me. Sure it was a lot of money, but I kept it on the kitchen table for a few days, not even looking at it. Part of me wasn't entirely sure he wasn't going to ask for it back. I'd seen a lot of cash in the past few years; it comes and goes quickly. Most of us, escorts that is, we make it, and then we spend it. We buy beauty products and new outfits. I even treated myself to a new car. Then we need to make it again. Then we spend it because we know we can make it again.

'The smart ones pay themselves a wage,' Nina once told me. Easier said than done.

With J, I kept my word and cancelled all my clients for the week. I saw him a few evenings later (he was busy with work). Lin picked me up again and we spent the best part of the drive to the city chatting. 'Mr J – he a good man!' Lin told me. 'He look after me!'

It was nice to hear J was good to his staff. He did seem like a lovely man, but the time off had given me food for thought. It was all a bit too good to be true. Even the movies aren't like this.

This time, we had sex (briefly) and went to dinner in a busy part of town where people went to be seen. He was still pushing for me to say yes, that I would live with him, that I would give everything up for him.

'But my business, darling. What do I tell my clients?'

'You tell them you are off the market. For good.'

And so it went on. The movie. Because that's what it felt like. Except I think, deep down, we both knew this wasn't real. I wanted to believe him, but I knew better than that. He wanted the fantasy. And I wanted to believe I wanted him, but again, I didn't.

It all ended as quickly as it began. I made the fatal error of texting him when I had clients trying to book me in for a few weeks' time. When I dared to question his 'deal', it seemed to push him over the edge.

You care more about your clients than me. It's over, he wrote back just two days after our first 'date'.

And that was it. I'd been virtually married and divorced in a week. I felt baffled by the whole drama. But of course, I'd been down a similar road a few times before.

So here was the danger in the world of private escorting – falling for the bullshit. Because as quickly as you could be picked as the cherry on top of the cake you could just as easily be discarded. The trick is, I soon learnt, not to take these promises to woo you away to a land of milk and honey too seriously.

Since J, there have been many, many more. A client took me out on his helicopter, where I drank champagne as we glided past Sydney Harbour Bridge at sunset, and landed in the bush, far from the city, amongst galloping wild horses and kangaroos. Admit it: who hasn't wanted to have sex in the back of a helicopter, the blades still whirring, a bottle of Moët propped against the seat? Another took me to the opera; the next client after that took me on his boat.

Having a driver drop me home is not unusual these days. My clients are mostly the type of men who have private drivers, and I always accept. I almost half-expect it now. The novelty has worn off. I don't even make conversation with the drivers any more.

Sometimes clients drive me home themselves – or at least to my suburb. One client recently insisted he take me in his brand new Porsche, even though my car was parked outside my unit in the city. He just wanted to hold my hands for that little bit extra. I didn't say anything. We both took comfort in that journey – the closeness, the faux intimacy. That he wasn't just a client, and I wasn't just an escort.

As I am writing this, I am also juggling appointments for next week. A 10 am with Steve, then a two-hour appointment with Jason. It's exciting, but something is missing. I can't deny that.

There is a part of me that longs for a normal life again, to be loved by a normal man, and to have a normal relationship. I know now that I had it before, but I didn't know what I had then. I had felt suffocated, and yearned for a different life. Now that I'm here and living it, sure, it's exciting. But my craving is for normality. I long for cuddles, not filthy sex. I want to be loved, not drooled over. I am getting sick of making other people happy and going home alone. There is a part of me that wants to pull my hair extensions out, let my pubes grow, and take off the make-up. To throw out the stockings and wear comfy tracksuits instead, or to find excitement in going to the movies with a boyfriend instead of meeting a stranger for a sexy rendezvous.

But Samantha's pull, her desire for wild, abandoned freedom, is harder.

I lie in bed sometimes and cry out for Rosie, my 55-kilo Rottweiler–Ridgeback cross, to get off the couch and come and sleep with me. Sometimes she obeys me, and I smile as I can hear her *pad pad pad* across the floorboards to my room. Her warm body that gently rises up and down with each snore almost makes me feel like I am with man. I throw her paw over me and snuggle into her chest. It only takes seconds for me to drift off, safe in her arms, feeling loved and protected.

Will I ever have a man in my bed again? Will I ever love? Will I ever decide it's time to stop this nonsense, this merry-go-round of texts, clients, sex, money, and repeat five times a week? Smokers have nicotine patches. What do hooked sex workers have?

When I started writing this book I thought I had the ending. I'll probably fall in love, that's a good place to end the book, I hoped secretly. Isn't that what happens? That's always the tried and tested formula isn't it, with sex workers. I did it, I fell in love, I got out. Not in this case. I did it, I'm doing it, I enjoy it. I am not capable of falling in love. Am I?

'I need a deadline extension,' I panicked to my agent. 'I don't know how this book is going to end.' I was still living it. Samantha was still alive. I wasn't any closer to an ending.

I'm still waiting.

I thought that it would be far more socially acceptable for me to come out as the author of this book as long as I had stopped working. As long as Samantha was gone, was old news. Something I did, someone I used to know. 'Oh yes, I used to do it. Oh no, not any more!' I imagined myself telling people when they asked. Somehow, that would be easier for people to swallow. I used to be a drug addict, I used to drink, I used to be a sex worker . . .

I stand corrected.

Love isn't going to happen as long as Samantha takes centre stage. It's just not. I can trick myself into thinking that the man I'm going to fall in love with is just around the corner. Any minute now someone is going to sweep me off my feet!

But in my grand old age comes wisdom. I've been down this road before. Falling in love isn't a fluke, it's a choice. You're only going to fall in love when these things happen:

1) You're open to falling in love.
2) It's the right time in your life.

The man is almost irrelevant. Sure, he'd have to have big arms, a good job, make me laugh, be kind. But there's no point having this man bump into me in the street corner with a Tiffany's box under my nose if I'm not in the right place. There's no point meeting him when I am not capable of love. And with Samantha taking all the attention, what chance does Amanda have?

I know I need to kill Samantha off if indeed it is love I am searching for. But I just can't do it – I haven't even tried yet. It's addictive and I'm the first to admit I'm hooked. 'Hello, my name is Amanda (or is it Samantha?) and I am addicted to being a call girl.'

It's a show and I get to star in it. I love getting dressed up. I love the thrill of meeting new men, someone new and mysterious whose story I don't know yet, someone who is going to get the best of me, and I'm certainly going to get the best of him. I'd miss these little frissons, the hour-long trailer clips of the real story. After all, you're not getting the beginning or the end, just the best bit somewhere in the middle.

I can be the sex siren. I enjoy being the seductress, not the wife. I enjoy clipping my suspender belt on every day, not an apron. I choose lace gloves over oven gloves any day. It's the passionate sex and the filthy text messages I like to receive. Not his credit card statements and his dry-cleaning.

But it comes at a price. I know that well. I go home alone at the end of every day. When I turned 40 I spent a beautiful day with my very best girlfriends, but I still woke up by myself the next day.

Just as I was coming to writing the end of this book, I was hit hard with pneumonia. It came out of nowhere and left me bedridden for a week. You know who surprised me? My clients.

My favourites called or texted every day and one even sent flowers. I was feeling so sorry for myself that I wept on the phone to Robert, a client from Brisbane whom I hadn't even met.

'Hey, you drink whisky?' he said, trying to cheer me up.

'No,' I croaked, my chest feeling like an elephant was sitting on it. Whisky . . . wasn't that the drink that made me sick in Italy all those years ago? I forget now . . .

'You should start. Half a bottle of whisky and a hot shower will sort you out, no problem,' he said brightly. 'Works for me every time! Try it!'

I started bawling.

'What's . . . sorry . . . did I say something wrong?'

I couldn't really talk. It wasn't just because I was in too much pain, I didn't know what to say. I hadn't even met this client. We'd been playing cat and mouse trying to arrange a meeting, and now my sickness had stuffed us around more. But this stranger was being so nice to me that it made me sad.

Where was my mum?

I put the phone down and had a good cry. His kindness was a little prod, a sharp reminder of what it was like having someone who cared. So that's what it felt like. Comforting. Safe. I hadn't felt those things in a while.

Being sick was like a purge for me. It was like someone was saying, 'Now sit down and rest! You've got a lot to think about.' And I did. As painful as it was, I thought about my parents.

A few times while I was lying there, I punched out an email. 'Dear Mum and Dad.' But when it was ready to send I pressed Delete instead.

I thought about the men in my life. The real ones. I hadn't been that nice to them, really. My coldness, my ability to disconnect, was a useful tool in Samantha's game but a hurtful one in real life. I cut people out of my life when I'd had enough. That's it, I'd decide somewhere along the line, I don't like you any more. Record your TV shows on *my* Foxtel IQ? Get out of my house. You want to date me? You want to get to know me? Please don't. I'm not that interesting. I'm a working girl. Please don't love me; don't even like me. Didn't you hear me? I'm a working girl now. Doesn't that put you off? It should.

Could I ever let anyone get close to me? Was it possible?

'You've never been in love before, have you?' a psychic asked me recently. Well, it wasn't so much a question – we both knew the answer.

'No,' I whispered, the tears falling fast onto my Tarot card. *Shut up Amanda, shut up shut up shut up.*

I tried to swallow but the lump in my throat hurt. It was sore. I didn't want to cry. Let me swallow my pain away.

'Amanda, it's okay to cry. Allow yourself to feel vulnerable, to feel sad, to feel loss,' she said quietly, taking my hand, which was shaking by now. Her skin was soft, like my mother's. 'Because, darling, if you don't start loving yourself, how can anyone else?'

Look, I really didn't want to go here. It's too deep. It's too personal. Let me stay light and bright and funny. I'm like a little colourful whirlwind, aren't I? You love hearing about how fun my life is. How exciting. How wild! Let me tell how wonderful it all is. I can do that! Let me tell you about the men, the money, the flash of a gold card, the clink of a champagne flute, kicking off my Louboutins and whoops, there goes my skirt!

And have I told you about the hotel rooms, the balconies, the view, where you were so high up you could touch the stars with your hands? Did I show you this bracelet he gave me? That smell? Oh that's my new perfume, Coco Noir, from Chanel – a gift of course!

I must tell you about that boat, that helicopter, that trip! The poor thing, he feels so unloved at home. His wife you see, she ignores him. Him! How can she not keep her hands off him? He's so lovely, isn't he? So *loveable*. I nuzzle in his neck and breath in his unique smell. What do you mean that smell isn't mine? His wife doesn't touch him any more! Don't look at me like that! It's me he comes to. It's me he desires. Oh, he's got a thing for my stockings – did you know he buys me a pair every time he sees me? The good ones, from Wolfords. No cheap crap for me, darling. First class all the way!

Oh, do excuse me, there goes my phone. Oh look! What do we have here? Another booking: *Hi Samantha, great profile. Free for dinner tonight? I do hope so . . . I'm staying at the Westin . . . does 8 pm suit? Tony.*

Another client.

Hi Tony . . .

Another story.

Come on Amanda, what's it to be? It's time to jump off now, baby. Jump off the ride. You've had your fun – boy! What fun you've had! Sure, you're worth the money but the right one won't have to pay a cent. You don't even want the money, do you, Amanda? You don't even count it. Are you ready for him, Amanda? Are you ready to fall in love? Are you ready to be loved? Come on baby, enough of this now. It's time, Amanda. It's time to be loved.

Hi Tony . . . perfect. Can't wait. Samantha X

THE AFTERMATH
WHAT HAPPENED NEXT TO
SAMANTHA X

And so it happened. The aftermath. The bloodshed. The 'coming out'. Former journalist reveals all! 'Tuck shop mum's double life as an escort' . . .

Gasp. Horror! A MOTHER, a 40-year-old, leaves her low-paid job as a respectable tabloid reporter and gets paid handsomely by the hour for *sex?* Whatever is the world coming to? Has she lost her marbles?

And to top it all off, she volunteers in the school canteen. Wait, *what?*

Escorts don't work in school canteens. They certainly don't have kids. Besides, most of us are monsters who walk around in a slunken stoop, only stopping to self-flagellate with our (shiny, black) leather whips for being such awful human beings. Beware, we walk among you. We shop at the same supermarkets and breathe the same air, too. Forget terrorists. It's hookers you need to worry about.

This is what surprised me so much about the whole media circus: the fact I worked once a fortnight in the tuck shop of my local primary school was what seemed to interest Australia the most.

I think of all the interesting questions journalists could have asked me, all the funny stories I could have told them, everything I've learnt about men and sex. Who are my celebrity clients? What are my best tricks? Could I talk about the married doctor who wanted me to bark like a Jack Russell on all fours? But no. What they wanted to know most about was my role as sausage roll and beef pie 'wrapper-upper' in the bloody school canteen. How did my 'other' job affect my work at the school? Was I still welcome there? (Yes, on the condition that I share my juicy stories with the other canteen mums). By the way, I'm a much better escort than I am tuck-shop assistant. I once made salad sandwiches out of the wilting brown lettuce leaves and egg shells from the compost bowl, having mistaken them for the real salad. But for Christmas my colleagues did receive pink and lacy Victoria's Secret G-strings, so I think all is forgiven . . .

Coming out was bigger than I thought it was going to be. Sure, I knew I would ruffle a few conservative, God-fearing feathers out there. I certainly didn't walk into the furnace with my eyes shut, thinking no one would give a hoot.

But what I did not expect was for the news to go global. For *The Sun* newspaper to do a big splash, or *The Daily Mail UK* to make me its headline story. I was even invited to LA to appear on a talk show. Seriously? I was hardly re-inventing the wheel: prostitution is, after all, the oldest profession.

Except, not so, as it would seem for 40-year-old escorts who are (bated breath, closed eyes, come on spit it out): *mothers*. The fact I had kids caused a torrent of vitriolic abuse spouting from the thinly pursed lips of apparently 'better' mothers than me who thought my role in society was awful, tutting my 'poor, poor' children and raging about what a terrible, selfish mother I was, and how because of my job, my kids would have to endure a life of misery, bullying and shame (probably from their own kids). I was a whore and a slut and an anti-feminist, and someone call DoCS now!

Oh – and that I was a selfish, narcissistic attention seeker who hungrily devoured every second of my 15 minutes of fame, deliciously licking my lips at the glory.

I just didn't think one iota about my kids, my parents and my ex.

Ouch.

Yes, I shed a few tears.

Then it was, 'Am I really that bad?' to my best friend Tab, Doris, my counsellor, and a few others.

But after that it became, 'They can all just fuck off!', to myself. Of course, I would never be rude, so instead responded very politely to a few of my online trolls. 'Thank you for your comments,' was my usual, restrained reply to a few women (and it was only women) who had gone to the bother of tracking my email address down, and telling me in great detail why I am a terrible person and how offended and disgusted they are by me.

Look, I won't pretend it wasn't awful. It wasn't exactly water off a duck's back. During those three or four days after my 'explosive revelations' on Seven's *Sunday Night* show, I barely left my house. (The kids were at their dad's and for now none the wiser to any of this online frenzy). Every morning, after

Rosie had jumped on my bed and licked my face to wake me up, the first thing I did was scroll through the news on my phone, looking for those dreaded words, 'Escort mum.' Every single day that week, my heart would sink and I'd feel sick in my tummy again, waiting patiently for the day to end and the story to become old news.

A good friend of mine turned up every morning with fruit salad, yoghurt, green juices and coffee. 'You've got to eat,' he'd say, unpacking the plastic bags. He even called throughout the day to see how I was.

'Terrible,' would be my usual whimper.

'Get a bit of mongrel about ya,' he eventually said. 'Come on, Amanda. Where's that feisty woman gone? Don't take this crap. These people don't know you.'

He was right. That night, as I washed my face and eased a cold flannel onto my puffy eyes, I looked in the mirror. Fuck them all. I knew who I was. The people who loved me knew who I was. I adored my kids, and my kids adored me. I was a good person, a good mum, a good friend. I needed to toughen up.

If these people had read my book, even just thumbed through the bits that didn't talk about cock, pussy and sexless marriages (or other things that clearly hit a nerve for them), they would have read about the emotional turmoil, the torture I faced daily about my job, my kids and my future.

They would have read that I disowned my family a good while before I came out, and that my issues with them stem from many years of hurt.

They would have read that my kids are the most important people in my life and I do my best every day to be the best mother I can be.

But I have learnt along this journey that your profession does not define you as a human, let alone a parent, and as long as kids get bundles of unconditional love, your trust and your time, they'll be okay.

And that, quite frankly, everyone else can get stuffed.

The most surprising reaction, though, was not my haters, but the kindness I received from absolute strangers. Their voices were louder. Their voices were smarter, more educated and balanced.

My website had over 90,000 hits from 154 countries in a few days, Australia, Brazil, America and the UK being the most intrigued. I even got emails from Mauritius, Serbia, Russia, France and Italy. People were writing in to me in their droves, wanting me to solve their love and sex issues, or simply congratulating me on my bravery, and, of course, most of them were asking to book an appointment with me.

Lots of women write to me too, asking for advice on how to become as escort, having thought about for many years, or how should they treat a man, or does their husband cheat (for example, what signs should they look for?).

A few write to me to say they have given up their boring accountancy or law job to become an escort. They want to thank me for going public and making them realise it was okay to like sex, and want to get paid for it. Escorts have written to me saying thank you for coming out and giving the industry an intelligent voice. Even some bosses of escort agencies and websites wrote to say 'Thanks, we love you!'

One woman wrote to me about growing up with her mother, who'd been a high-class escort. The woman had only admiration and adoration for her mother, and she was never bullied. That email in particular I'll hold close to my heart.

So every time I read comments like this on my Facebook page: 'You're disgusting, you WHORE, you SLUT AMANDA GOFF!!!! YOU DESERVE TO LOSE YOUR CHILDREN AND GET AIDS' from a lady wearing a footy jumper and missing a front tooth, I can easily delete and ignore them. There are other letters to cherish, like this one: (an actual email I received, printed word for word.)

Dear Samantha,

I purchased your book yesterday and found it incredibly inspiring and your inner strength wonderful. As a professional can I say that every profession has its high and low points/days and, although those that can be experienced in your work can be extreme, you are a model citizen in the way you maintain your ethics and care for others around you. I am a divorcee of almost ten years and have recently, for the first time, met with a professional like yourself (I guess that helps back up the statistics in your book) and I was fortunate to find a true lady like yourself and enjoyed a very special dinner date. Friends transcend all and the true friends you describe in your book sound wonderful. I am sure that you will continue to do what you believe gives you the best opportunities to be the best mother and I am sure that under your guidance your children will grow into wonderful adults. In the book I read many insightful and inspiring words for anyone, in any form of profession, and I encourage you to continue to take your life along the path that you believe is for you. I have not met you but I am proud of you and wish you every happiness and success.

Happy Christmas
Sincerely
John

Honestly, what a lovely message. The fact that people were taking time out of their busy lives to write to me was really touching. I set up the Samantha X Facebook page, and my own website (www.samanthax.com.au) and received hundreds of messages from strangers all over the world wanting to be friends. Even beyond Facebook, men, women, Psychology students, professors and sometimes the odd celebrity have reached out to me.

I get stopped in the street and congratulated or thanked – here in Sydney and interstate. I was once actually in my car, sitting in traffic, when a man next to me practically put his head through my window.

'Oh you're that lady!' he beamed. 'That very brave lady. Good for you, Samantha!'

'Mum, who was that?' asked my son, his eyes momentarily lifting up from his iPad.

But as anyone who has been in the public eye, albeit briefly, would know, it is the offers of cold meats from strangers that mean the most. I was walking near my home with the kids when a man spotted me. 'Wait here, Miss Samantha!' he said excitedly before climbing into his van. He emerged holding an enormous leg of ham.

'I loved your book,' he said, passing me the meat. 'The world needs more people like you around. Please, take this, and enjoy it with your family.'

I, for once, was almost lost for words. 'Thank you?' I was not quite sure what to do with the bone of pink fleshy meat.

'Mum, don't eat it, it could be poisoned,' hissed my eight-year-old as he clutched my hand tightly.

Suffice to say, Rosie the Rottweiler, Georgie the Jack Russell, and our two kittens, Fluffy and Ginger, enjoyed ham for weeks after that. Those animals are *really* happy I went public.

You want to know what my kids have been exposed to since coming out? That. No teasing at the playground; no name calling. I'm sure there are people who think I'm awful, who probably bitch and gossip about me behind my back. But they are smart enough not to say it to my face and even smarter not to say anything in front of or to my kids. And woe betides the person who thinks it's a good idea to bring it up with my children.

Sure, the kids have asked questions about my book. I have told them it is about sex and it is for adults, and one day when they are old enough, I will explain it to them. I have also told them to tell me if anyone mentions it at school, and I check with them regularly.

'No, Mum, no one cares,' said my son once, exasperated after a little prying question from me. 'No one cares what you do, get over it. Can we go to the skate park?'

His little snap at me was, if anything, a welcome relief.

So when a journalist phoned me to ask how I was coping with the fallout, waiting (hoping?) for me to break down sobbing, 'Forgive me I beg of you!' I just smiled and said, 'Fine, thanks.'

'No regrets?'

'None.'

'Really?'

'Really.'

'What about your ex-colleagues, the journalists?'

'What about them?'

'Some of them have been saying how shocked they are, worried for you . . . Have you been reading the press?'

'Not really. It's irrelevant. It's not my day-to-day life. They are entitled to their opinion, of course.'

'Your ex-husband?'

'Yes?'

'He said –'

And so it went on.

Okay, my ex. Did he know? 'Course he did. He knew for yonks. Didn't like it, didn't want me to do it. But it wasn't a shock, there was no surprise, no 'Now I have to tell our children.' Do people really think I would write a book about being a call girl and go on telly, and not think to mention it to my ex and family?

I could tell you about the photographer on a moped who ambushed my ex and the kids one morning before school, the day after my television interview had aired.

I could tell you about the ear bashing said photographer got from my ex, and how those very words were twisted into a great headline, something along the lines of 'Ex-husband of Escort Mum breaks his silence: *"This is a disgrace . . . Now I am going to have to tell the kids . . ."*' I won't go into too much detail.

But even I had to hand it to the editor. When you can't get the truth, twist it. The public don't care! God knows I did it enough times when I was a reporter. Sod the truth: it's a great story!

One thing I did take away from all of this – thank God I left journalism and all its scrappy, unscrupulous morals. Give me the ethics and class of the sex industry any day. Seriously.

The whole situation was pretty ironic. Me, getting lynched for having a terrible disgusting shameful job like escorting and being honest about it, when I did far worse, morally and ethically (not to mention illegal), during my time as a reporter.

As with sex workers, we aren't all bonkers. And not all reporters are scrappy. One in particular, is very good. Sarrah Le Marquand asked me to write an opinion piece for *The Daily Telegraph*. I respect and trust her, so I thought that, after five days of being in the very public firing line, it was time to respond to some of my critics. She printed my piece and hopefully, just hopefully, it shut up a few people. I've reproduced it below.

————————

If any day was going to be tough this week, it was going to be the first day back at the tuck shop. What would be waiting for me, I wondered as I nervously walked through the playground. A gang of angry mums baying for my blood? Would I find my victimised children sobbing in a crumpled heap? Or – from what some people in this country clearly feel would be an adequate punishment for me – a wooden cross ready for my crucifixion?

It was, dare I say it, just another ordinary day. 'Amanda, love, fill up the paper bags with tomato sauce, and remember Dylan from 1B likes two with his meat pie,' said Joan, the head chef at our primary school's canteen. She barely even looked up.

'Good week, darling?' asked Julie, the 2IC, giving me a quick peck on my cheek. 'Saw you on the telly. Good for you. Bought the book, can't wait to read it. When you've done the sauce, can you butter the jacket potatoes?'

Hang on. Haven't I just this week brought shame and disrepute to my community, my family and myself? Haven't I single handedly taken feminism backwards 10,000 years, wasn't I the sole person responsible for all the married men in this country straying, and oh, of course, how could I forget – wrecking my children's lives in the process?

Seemingly not, according to the people I care about the most: the school mums, my local community and, most importantly, my kids.

Because life for *us* this week has been as ordinary as ever. Yep, when I think about the endless cups of tea I've drunk, the tracksuit pants I've lived in and the cat I had to take to the vet, life has been pretty boring.

I've had a few panicked phone calls from worried friends. 'God Amanda, have you seen the online stuff? Don't read it, it's terrible,' a friend panted breathlessly as I was stirring my tea one gloomy afternoon, wondering when this rain was ever going to stop.

'I'm just wondering how you are coping with this vicious nasty stuff? God some people are just so evil . . .' said another girlfriend.

Can you see where I am going with this?

As the keyboard warriors are gleefully foaming at the mouth furiously tapping angry words like 'whore' and 'slut' and 'selfish bad mother' in a topic that has apparently 'divided a nation', (someone else's words, not mine), I can't help but wonder, as I get on with my rather dull and normal existence, am I the only bloody person in this country who is mildly bemused by this hysterical circus?

Let me set a few things straight. Here are some questions some people have raised, which I think rightly need answering. I've addressed them all in my book, but for those of you who are too disgusted to buy it (not many of you according to the recent sales figures), I'll say them here.

WHY DID I GO PUBLIC?

Believe it or not I didn't wake up and think, 'Hmm, bored today. I know! I'll out myself!' This was a very hard decision for me, as my publicist, agent, friends, and counsellor know. I have been a journalist for 20 years, and a sneaky one at that. I've hidden in bushes, illegally hacked phones and chased celebrities down the street. If I wrote my book under a pseudonym, you can bet your bottom dollar some triumphant reporter would one day turn up on my doorstep. The people who are important in my life have known for months what I do and we still get invited over for tea. I am not ashamed of myself, they are not ashamed to know me, and my kids are popular and well-loved. So rather live in nail-biting fear at one day someone outing me, like they did with Belle De Jour, I'd rather own it. It's just how I roll.

I'M A BAD AND SELFISH MOTHER.

I'm getting a bit sick of this one. I completely 110 per cent agree that our decisions can affect and damage our kids. I think my ex and I separating would have had a major effect on my eldest, who was four at the time. I think back to when we used to fight and I dread to think how many door slams he heard. If you scream at your kids all day, get constantly stoned or drunk, abuse them, neglect them, hit them, sexually abuse them, and put them down then yes, you will damage your kids, absolutely no question about it. But do I think being an escort damages kids? Well, let me put it this way. If you were a scientist, testing on defenceless animals all day, would that damage your kids? If you worked for a tobacco company building guns or nuclear weapons, would that damage your kids? Or if you worked at a fast

273

food outlet, pumping processed food into the mouths of our youth; would that damage your kids?

Some need to swindle deals or turn a blind eye to shady business deals. Some, God forbid, are parking officers. Are they damaging their kids? We do all sorts of things to make ends meet. We are entitled to do the jobs we want to do, or need to do, because as an adult, that is our right. Professions do not define our parenting skills. Our children do not have to *approve* of our choices. My children certainly would not have approved of our divorce, or many of the choices both their father and I have made and will continue to make. But it's not their life. It's not up to them. What children need is unconditional love, stability, trust, nurturing and your time. I hope my children grow up to be non-judgmental, open-minded, authentic and honest adults. I want them to show kindness and compassion to others and be the ones to come to the aid of someone crying in the playground, not kick him in the ankles for being weak. Those are the children I am proud to be the mother of. I can't see my kids ever bullying someone or deliberately hurting others with cruel words. It's just not the way their dad and I have brought them up. I can't protect them from the savage society we live in; I can only give them the tools to deal with judgmental narrow-minded people. So far, the only thing we had to deal with at school this week was my son getting hit on the head with a soccer ball which caused a few tears. So, while I appreciate your concern, my kids are fine, thank you very much. How are yours?

AM I ANTI-FEMINIST?
Let's clarify one thing: I have never said women should be tied to a vacuum cleaner, wearing a sexy maid's outfit while

their precious husbands are out making money. Men, of course, are not the only breadwinners. I wasn't talking about money. I was talking about *needs*. Men are men. They do manly stuff. Women are nurturers. You can still be a feminist and *feminine*. What I meant to say, but probably didn't come across well on a high-pressure (and edited) TV interview, was, why not transfer some of that nurturing we women are so good at on our husbands? And for the record, a woman who proudly spouts on about feminism, before calling another 'sister' a whore and a slut is hypocritical and lacks class. Am I anti-feminist? Not at all. I am anti-abuse, anti-rudeness, anti-bullying, anti-homophobic, anti-racist and anti-trolling. My favourite words this week are integrity and kindness.

SEX.
Looks like we've run out of space. For discussion next time!

———————

Since going public, I was absolutely inundated with requests. Hundreds of men (and women) from all over the world wanted to book me. I even put my prices up to $1000 an hour: $6000 a night. I could have made a million dollars if I had seen every person who asked.

But – as always – I remained picky (mental health over dollars any day). Most enquiries I politely declined. Photos of naked penises – no thanks. Six pack abs – maybe. Photos of you and the wife? Um . . . what?

Manners and respect secured bookings. Naked cock and arrogance would result in getting your number blocked.

I was seen as a 'celebrity' escort. A few clients said things like, 'I can't believe I am here lying with *you!*' But my all-time favourite was, 'It is so refreshing to see you have cellulite on your thighs.'

A security guard at the airport told me I was 'a naughty, naughty girl' as he scanned my body for God knows what (explosive dildos?), and a very sweet girl in a lingerie shop smiled and said, 'You are just as nice in person as you are on TV,' as she popped my G-strings into a bag.

What was interesting is that I attracted a new kind of client – a man who had never seen an escort before, but had seen me on TV and thought they would give it a go. Maybe they were surprised that escorts could actually string a sentence together and didn't appear to have needle marks on their arms.

'I watched your TV interview with my wife,' a boyishly handsome husband told me, taking his shirt off. 'She thought it was disgusting and asked me what I thought. "Oh she's terrible," I told her, but inside I was making a mental note to call you in a few weeks.'

It wasn't the first time I had heard that. One man flew from Miami to take me out for dinner every single night for a week. Another told me that while his wife and her friends were discussing my story, he tiptoed off to make an appointment. Another, on holiday in Sydney, sneaked off, while his wife was shopping at Westfield, to receive a massage and give me oral sex. His colleagues at the bank had been looking at my website when he felt the need to make an appointment to 'see what the fuss was all about.'

So business is booming. But, like I've said before, my job is not so much about sex as it is about communication and intimacy. One client told me, 'I'm going to be one of those clients that wants to talk, sorry,' and then proceeded to pour his heart out about his failed marriage.

Another confessed his wife had been cheating and asked what he should do.

Another had lost his wife to cancer and just wanted a warm body to hold as he wept.

My job has always been more about the talk than the sex. I had a 17-year-old school boy email me and ask me for tips on talking to women. I've had women in Brazil ask me to mentor them in how to swap their careers from HR to hooker . . . and so it goes on.

I have set up a Q & A page on my website so people can ask questions, where I personally reply and try to help. And great news! I am also now also the sex editor of *Penthouse* magazine, where I combine two of my loves: sex and writing. Readers send me questions about the size of their dicks, or confusion over the G spot to what to do if their wife cheats and I get to do what I do best – listen, help and heal – clothes ON this time. Penthouse definitely does not pay me $1000 an hour, but the job is just as rewarding. I have no degree in psychology, but my experience with men on an emotional and intimate level means far more than sitting on a plastic chair in a stuffy lecture hall learning about theories.

Samantha X? Her time must be running out, right? Tick tock, tick tock. Because I can't be Samantha X forever, can I? I am going to have to 'grow up and be normal' aren't I? Swap my stilettos for sensible. Suspender belts for superannuation. I am going to have a relationship, fall in love, and live happily ever after. *Won't I?*

My time as an escort is coming to an end. It is. My lease expired on my unit in the city, and I decided not to renew it.

I felt sad as I packed up – my stockings draped over chairs, my pearl necklace hanging over the bed post. When I closed the door for the final time, I knew it symbolised the end of something. Not just the pretty unit with water views – sure, I'll miss that and the laughter that radiated from inside. But I knew that I wouldn't get another unit. I didn't want to. I don't want to. I've met a few nice men that I would date, but I can't, because Samantha X is afraid of love.

I am sick of being afraid.

I am sick of sleeping alone.

I am sick of Samantha X.

But bigger than that, I am scared. I am scared I will never stop. Or that the fun ends and serious life begins. I swap controversy for convention. That scares me more.

One day I will lie on my death bed and, taking my last gasp, as my lungs bubble away and my heartbeat takes its last few flutters, I will think back to the whirlwind of hotels, green $100 notes and panting men. I will think back to this book and the beautiful strangers who reached out to me in support.

What will my epitaph say? 'Samantha X meant well'? 'Samantha X loved sex'?

'Bury me in my Louboutins,' I'll whisper hoarsely to my kids as I clutch their hands weakly.

But for now, this very second, the stilettos stay on. Lacy gloves replace oven gloves. Corsets over comfort.

Samantha X will retire one day. She will. Soon. Sooner than you think!

Honest.

Acknowledgements

If it wasn't for my dear friends persuading me to jot down my stories as and when they were occurring, this book probably would have stayed in my head. You know who you are – so thank you, ladies.

This book also wouldn't have been possible without the constant encouragement and support from my wonderful literary agent, Tara Wynne at Curtis Brown, my publisher, the lovely (and scarily intelligent) Alison Urquhart, and my patient editor, Elena Gomez – both from Random House Australia.

While it turned sour at the end, I do want to nod my head at the staff and girls at The Bordello. I'm not sure 'thank you' is fitting in this case, but I often think back fondly to the emotional, thought-provoking, eye-opening and (almost) always hilarious, time. It's not an easy job, but you do it well.

Thank you to Nina, my old madam, for her hilarious descriptions and for easing me into the sex industry, and Namaste to the Queensland retreat for allowing me to miss the morning hikes to write (when I was really asleep).

Writing a book as honest as this wasn't easy. I have spent many sleepless nights worrying about my children, my life and my reputation. But together with my wonderful counsellor, Doris, who kept me sane when I was feeling anything but, the school mums and dads, my friends and my local community who know me and (hopefully) love me for who I am – your support has helped me on this journey more than you could ever know. Thank you.

And of course, how could I not thank my sweet, kind and gorgeous clients, who think spending time with me is something special. I think each and every one of you is special too.

Lots of love,

Samantha X